JUMP START AUTOPHAGY

ACTIVATE Your Body's **CELLULAR HEALING** Process
to Reduce Inflammation, Fight Chronic Illness
and Live a Longer, Healthier Life

MELISSA MAYER

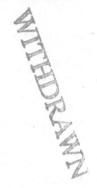

D1397584

Published in the United States by:
ULYSSES PRESS
P.O. Box 3440
Berkeley, CA 94703
www.ulyssespress.com

ISBN: 978-1-61243-938-9
Library of Congress Control Number: 2019942138

Printed in the United States by Kingery Printing Company
10 9 8 7 6 5 4 3 2 1

Acquisitions editor: Casie Vogel
Managing editor: Claire Chun
Project editor: Renee Rutledge
Proofreader: Jessica Benner
Indexer: S4Carlisle Publishing Services
Front cover design: Ashley Prine
Artwork: © Djem/shutterstock.com
Interior design and layout: what!design @ whatweb.com
Production editor: Jake Flaherty

NOTE TO READERS: This book has been written and published strictly for informational and educational purposes only. It is not intended to serve as medical advice or to be any form of medical treatment. You should always consult your physician before altering or changing any aspect of your medical treatment and/or undertaking a diet regimen, including the guidelines as described in this book. Do not stop or change any prescription medications without the guidance and advice of your physician. Any use of the information in this book is made on the reader's good judgment after consulting with his or her physician and is the reader's sole responsibility. This book is not intended to diagnose or treat any medical condition and is not a substitute for a physician.

This book is independently authored and published and no sponsorship or endorsement of this book by, and no affiliation with, any trademarked brands or other products mentioned within is claimed or suggested. All trademarks that appear in ingredient lists and elsewhere in this book belong to their respective owners and are used here for informational purposes only. The author and publisher encourage readers to patronize the quality brands mentioned and pictured in this book.

For my family

CONTENTS

CHAPTER 13: RECIPES TO BOOST AUTOPHAGY 113

CHAPTER 14: CONCLUSION 124

INTRODUCTION

JINKIES, YOU'RE OLD

Age happens to everyone. Things get harder. Your body starts to look and feel a bit less like yours and a pinch more like your parents' (*oh, god*). Maybe you have a benchmark birthday approaching, or you've reached the point where you have second thoughts before taking risks you once embraced. Perhaps you've been around long enough to see chinks in the armor of your youthful invincibility, or you could almost swear you heard the unnerving shuffle of the Reaper (just getting acquainted with your address, no big deal).

The glib maxim "aging is better than the alternative" may be technically true, but it certainly doesn't soothe the angst as you leave your relatively health-safe years for those more medically fraught. If you have relatives or friends who have faced health challenges—or if you have already stared down the barrel of a health crisis or chronic illness—those worries might show up even earlier. Even if you feel great right now, the truth is you want to stay that way.

There's good news: Science is unraveling the intricacies of autophagy—a cellular renovation and recycling program happening inside your cells right now—that promises to change the way you age. Thanks to autophagy, your cells and tissues boast an incredible turnover rate. Imagine this: Your cells degrade and replace every single protein in your body about every 60 days, renewing your cellular machinery and protecting against damage that shows up when those proteins build up.[1] Autophagy also targets other threats to your health, like pathogens, old organelles (the subunits within a cell), and abnormal cell contents.

It's an "enormously hot field in biology," opines autophagy pioneer Yoshinori Ohsumi, who won the Nobel Prize for his work in 2016 and sparked a flurry of excitement about the disease-fighting cell program among researchers from a wide range of fields.[2] The volume of new research on the topic is so staggering that, between writing the first word of this introduction and typing the last period in the conclusion, thousands of brand-spanking-new peer-reviewed papers hit the scientific journals. At times, writing this book has felt like standing in the middle of an avalanche, nerdily talking about snow mechanics while buried up to the chin.

And all this intensity is for good reason. Understanding the nuts and bolts of autophagy heralds the development of new treatments for some of the most feared diseases that come with age—things like cancer and Alzheimer's disease. It means stretching the average human life span without sacrificing good health. There's no doubt that autophagy is the science to watch right now, but you don't have to observe from the sidelines. There are actionable things you can do today to tip the odds in your favor.

---

1   Yoshinori Ohsumi. "Historical Landmarks of Autophagy Research," *Cell Research* 24 (2014): 9–23. https://doi.org/10.1038/cr.2013.169.

2   Ohsumi, "Historical Landmarks of Autophagy Research," 9–23.

Use this book to gain a deeper understanding of what's going on in your cells and learn to tap into a crucial stress mechanism that has evolved in a wide range species—autophagy—that may help your body age successfully. Living your best life isn't just about surviving as long as you can; it's about protecting your health so you can enjoy the life you have built.

CHOOSE YOUR OWN ADVENTURE

To geek out about what autophagy is, how the science unfolded, and what might be on tap in the near future, head to Part I.

To learn about how autophagy protects against specific age-related diseases, flip to Part II.

If you prefer to jump right to autophagy-enhancing techniques you can use right now, consider yourself cordially invited to Part III.

A QUICK NOTE

It's important to remember that while the underlying science is old enough to collect social security, the potential applications of autophagy are still emerging. Researchers are on the knife's edge of monetizing autophagy via drug development and personalized treatment options. Science this new relies first on animal model studies (yeast and worms and rats and monkeys, oh my) and then turns to human clinical trials, which are considerably more complicated.

It makes sense to catch the autophagy bug and DIY it a bit; after all, it's exciting! However, Debbie Downer, version Velma here to remind you that oversimplifying or jumping to conclusions is jeepers-level spooky, gang. Just because ideas are connected doesn't mean one causes the other. Or, in science-and-philosophy-speak, correlation does not imply causation. That's the goal here—to decant the science and the possibilities for your pleasure with the important caveat that you only know what you know when you know it. Which is basically a decent life philosophy.

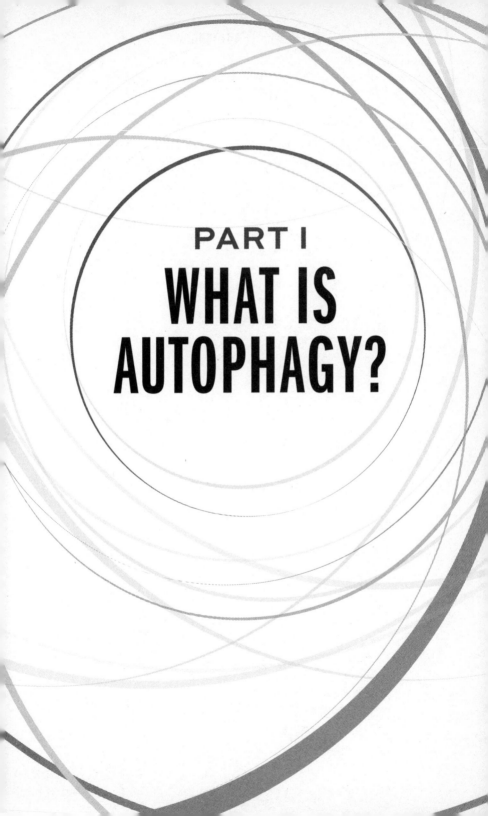

PART I
WHAT IS AUTOPHAGY?

CHAPTER 1

HOW AUTOPHAGY WORKS

TIME MACHINE TO ELEMENTARY BIOLOGY

You probably remember the fallout even decades later. You knew your science fair project was coming up but just couldn't deal, so you ignored it until an adult in charge, horrified by your life choices, discovered the assignment scrap in the bottom of your backpack...the day before it was due. The stress level surged, and your reasonable options were few, thanks to the now-impossible deadline. The only viable choice was the old standby: a cell model.

Maybe you sat up all night forming organelles out of clay and pressing them into a cytoplasm shell, topped off with handmade labels on toothpicks (bam, done). Perhaps you were more daring (or had a more creative parent) and suspended fruits or candies in gelatin for a science-meets-snack project. (Side note: Please, for the love of all that is holy, don't send one of these to school for your own kids. It attracts ants. And somebody is going to stick their finger in it, setting off a drama spiral that makes everybody late for recess. Signed, a former science teacher.)

Regardless of your medium, you probably still remember the big, important organelles (looking at you, nucleus, over there hogging all the cell biology glory). But you might not remember much about the rather boring-appearing, roundish blob you stuck near the cell membrane: the lysosome. Yet this relatively neglected organelle plays a powerful role in one of your body's most important processes: autophagy.

WHAT EVEN IS A LYSOSOME?

Lysosomes are round organelles enclosed by membranes. This membrane is an important barrier between the lysosome and the cytoplasm (the thick solution that fills each cell), since the interior of the lysosome is super acidic, which is a handy way to be if your job is taking things apart. These are your body's recycling centers, and they are chock-full of hydrolytic enzymes, which use water to break things down.

All the stuff your cells don't want hanging around—misfolded or malfunctioning proteins, old organelles or biomolecules, even bits of viruses or bacteria that might make you sick—get a direct ticket to the lysosome. Literally. Running through the cell's cytoplasm, a matrix of protein fibers called the cytoskeleton gives the cell its shape and organization. Some fibers act as tethers, anchoring organelles in place. Other fibers, called microtubules, form tracks around the cell. Cell transporters use these tracks to carry rejected cargo from other parts of the cell right to the lysosome's door.

Once there, the lysosome's enzymes break down the unwanted cell components. Some parts are reused to build new cell components, which conserves the cell's energy since spare parts are free. Some cargo is broken down even further and burned for energy. And some cargo is just tossed in the trash pile and destroyed, or taken to the cell membrane and pushed out of the cell.

ENTER AUTOPHAGY

Of course, all that unwanted stuff doesn't just hop on the train and head to the lysosome on its own. A tightly regulated (and pretty universal among organisms—thanks, evolution!) cell process called the autophagy lysosomal pathway handles that. This is a stress response, so while baseline-level autophagy happens all the time in your cells, stress caused by dwindling nutrients or oxygen sends out signals (code red! starving!) that kick it into high gear.

The cell responds to the stress signal by building a double-membrane bubble—called a vesicle or autophagosome, if you're fancy—ready to load up and transport unwanted cargo. The vesicle transporter engulfs that cargo—either unselectively because it just happens to be in the neighborhood or selectively seeking it out by mechanisms still under review—like a hungry blob and moves it into the cytoplasm using those microtubule tracks. Eventually, the vesicle fuses with the lysosome, where the cargo is unloaded, stripped for parts, and degraded.

Autophagy (as in the ancient Greek terms *auto* + *phagy*) literally means "self-devouring" because, when viewed through a microscope, it appears that the vesicle transporter swallows the unwanted cell contents.

WHY AUTOPHAGY MATTERS

As you age, unwanted material—especially those misfolded or otherwise malfunctioning proteins—accumulates in your cells and eventually causes disease. This is because the precise way a protein folds into a three-dimensional shape—its conformation—enables that protein to do its specific job. This is especially true for enzymes, a class of proteins that make the chemical reactions that keep you alive (like metabolism) work. These proteins connect with their target molecules like a lock fitting with a key. Misfolded proteins are terrible locks; the keys just won't fit.

The way a protein folds is determined much earlier in the process. To build a protein, the cell receives instructions from the nucleus so it can "translate" a string of base pairs copied from the DNA into a chain of amino acids, which will eventually fold into a functional protein. A change to even one amino acid—say, leaving one out or substituting it for another—can wreck a protein, rendering it nonfunctional and even directly causing diseases like cystic fibrosis or sickle cell anemia.

Those misfolded proteins cause problems over time, too. They can build up in your cells, forming the tangles or toxic clumps seen in neurodegenerative conditions, such as Alzheimer's disease, Creutzfeldt-Jakob disease, Parkinson's disease, and type 2 diabetes.

To understand the sort of function autophagy performs, consider the current theory on Alzheimer's disease. One of the primary features of the devastating neurodegenerative illness is neurofibrillary tangles of tau proteins in the brain cells. These proteins normally act like support beams for the nerve cells, giving them structure and helping them perform their jobs. However, abnormal or damaged tau proteins can't function properly and instead collapse into tangles. The precise mechanisms behind these tangles is still unclear; in fact, scientists very recently proposed a new mathematical model for how these clumps form and even spread among brain cells.[3]

Your cells don't just sit back and allow misfolded (or otherwise problematic) proteins to stack up. Most of these proteins, as well as other unwanted cellular matter, are tagged for destruction and routed through the cell's recycling machinery. This is autophagy, crucial for prolonging your health span and enabling you to age successfully.

GENES, GENES, GENES

The human genome contains somewhere between 20,000 and 25,000 genes, which are the basic unit of heredity.[4] Those genes are segments of paired nitrogen base molecules (plus a sugar and a phosphate) whose sequence codes for specific proteins, like a DNA recipe. Some genes are small, consisting of a couple hundred DNA bases, and some are ginormous at over 2 million bases. Each nucleus-containing cell in your body holds a full copy of your genome (which varies from the genomes of other humans by less than 1 percent!). If you were to place all that DNA end to end and stretch it out, it would cover the diameter of the sun...twice. Yet it fits inside your body, inside the nucleus of your cells, thanks to its super-twisted helical structure and the fact that it condenses into chromosomes.

Many of your genes serve as blueprints that tell your body how to build specific proteins. Other than water, proteins are the most abundant thing in your body, and they play a wide range of roles to keep

---

3 Carol J. Huseby et al. "The Role of Annealing and Fragmentation in Human Tau Aggregation Dynamics," *Journal of Biological Chemistry* 294, no. 13 (2019): 4728–37. https://doi.org/10.1074/jbc.RA118.006943.

4 National Institutes of Health, Genetics Home Reference. "What Is a Gene?" US Department of Health and Human Services, May 14, 2019. https://ghr.nlm.nih.gov/primer/basics/gene.

you alive and functioning. Researchers have uncovered approximately a gazillion genes and proteins (okay, not really, but a whole freaking lot) involved in autophagy across all research species. When it comes to humans, the HUGO Gene Nomenclature Committee currently lists 33 *autophagy-related genes* (*ATGs*).[5] The Human Autophagy Database (HADb), which is a public cache trying to keep up with the burgeoning literature, lists 232 genes that play direct or indirect roles in the autophagy lysosomal pathway.[6]

KEEPING IT ALL IN BALANCE

One of the central themes in cell biology is that organisms need to maintain homeostasis; that is, a stable, life-sustaining internal landscape built by constant tweaks and adjustments to keep it just right for survival. In a word, balance.

A straightforward example of homeostasis is your comfy normal body temperature of 98.2°F. This average temp isn't really real; it varies based on lots of factors, including your age, the flux of your hormones, the time of day—and even things like your sex assignment and race. In fact, your actual "normal" temperature is more like a fingerprint, which means your threshold for fever is not the same as your partner's or best friend's.

Still, whatever your normal is, your body works hard to stay there. Sensors that make up your central nervous system continuously gather temperature data and send it to your hypothalamus, a pebble-sized area near the base of your brain. The hypothalamus uses that data

---

5   HUGO Gene Nomenclature Committee. "Autophagy-Related Gene Group." https://www
.genenames.org/data/genegroup/#!/group/1022.

6   Guy Berchem and the Laboratory of Experimental Cancer Research. Human Autophagy
Database. Luxembourg Institute of Health. http://www.autophagy.lu/index.html.

to regulate your body temperature by kicking up sweat production and widening your blood vessels if you are too warm, causing you to shiver and altering your metabolism, and constricting those blood vessels when you get too cold. The whole shebang is meant to keep you at just the right temperature, no matter what goes on around you (or inside you).

The opposite of homeostasis is dysregulation, or being out of balance. When your body temperature becomes dysregulated, it can rise high enough to cause brain damage or kill you, or drop so low you develop hypothermia or can't fight off fungal infections (that last bit is the reason mammals edged out other vertebrates after the dinosaurs were wiped out—the warm-blooded body temperature system was one advantage against fungal infection in an environment marked by a changing climate and fungus blooms).

When it comes to your autophagy lysosomal pathway, the recurring motif is also balance. Your genes and signaling pathways (especially those called PKA, AMPK, and mTOR) work together to regulate autophagy such that it turns on precisely when it should. What's more, the whole point of autophagy is to maintain cellular homeostasis, or a steady state in your cells. When this falls apart, the resulting imbalance can lead to things like cancer and neurodegeneration. Dysregulated autophagy leads to disease, plain and (not so) simple.

CHAPTER 2

A QUICK AND DIRTY HISTORY

ONCE UPON A TIME IN JAPAN

When Yoshinori Ohsumi recounted his childhood for his Nobel Prize biographical sketch, he described endless days tramping through hills and paddies, combing streams and the sea for insects and plants to add to his collections, and poring over science books carefully curated by his elder brother, who was away at college. The image he painted feels idyllic—almost mystical—to a reader scrolling through the story of a bucolic boyhood against the backlit glow of an iPhone. The note of curiosity and exploration he describes of his early days would follow Ohsumi throughout his schooling and career, guiding his choices and leading his discoveries.

So, too, would the harsher specters of his youth. Ohsumi was born in Japan at the tail end of World War II, a time when the entire country was gripped by poverty and food scarcity. The son of an academic, Ohsumi recalls himself as a weak child, sickly with malnourishment.

And he wasn't the only sick person in his family. His mother, Shina, contracted tuberculosis after his birth and spent nearly a decade bed- and pain-ridden.

And this image—of a naturally curious young boy watching his mother suffer in a plaster cast, the bones of her spine disintegrating from spinal caries—grabs the spotlight in the researcher's biographical statement. Fortunately for the Ohsumi family, a care package from scientist friends in Hawaii changed the trajectory of Shina's life—and her son's. Inside that package lay a cutting-edge treatment, a cure for the disease that had robbed Ohsumi's mother of her health and a young boy of his mother. That cure? Antibiotics.

A CURIOUS DISCOVERY

The curiosity that marked Ohsumi's childhood pulled him toward the emerging scientific fields of cell biology and molecular biology, and guided his choices as a young researcher. During his postgraduate studies, Ohsumi noticed a peculiar layer of white matter in the centrifuge tubes he was processing. Intrigued by what this could be and otherwise unimpressed with the results of the actual research he was performing, Ohsumi glanced at the white stuff under the microscope and saw highly purified vacuoles.

These organelles were considered nothing more than trash compartments and were uninteresting to other researchers at the time, but the sight stuck with Ohsumi. He began a pet project exploring the vacuole membrane, which he says his colleagues probably thought a weird study subject. Soon, he uncovered the mechanisms the organelle uses to actively transport molecules across the membrane.

When he achieved an associate professorship, which came with his very own (albeit modest) lab, Ohsumi kept with the vacuole. He cultivated a line of yeast cells without proteases—the enzymes the vacuole uses to degrade proteins—so that the cell matter digested by the vacuole might stick around long enough to be visible, even under Ohsumi's basic microscope. The intrepid researcher starved the cells he scored from a colleague and, within half an hour, saw dramatic things. He couldn't tear his eyes away from the view under his lens; the vacuoles teemed with rapidly moving spheres.

Ohsumi took his work to colleagues with powerful electron microscopes and described the images he left with as "overwhelmingly beautiful."[7] Those zooming spheres were autophagic bodies, and these images unlocked the membrane dynamics of autophagy, at least in yeast cells. They also pushed Ohsumi toward the next step of his research: uncovering what genes and proteins play a role in autophagy. This work would consume the next eight years of Ohsumi's career. Ultimately, thanks to a collaboration with Ohsumi's wife and fellow scientist Mariko Nakazawa's lab and the serendipitous sequencing of the full yeast genome, Ohsumi's lab identified the major autophagy genes, called the *ATG* genes.

Even Ohsumi, who comes across in his biographical statement as carefully self-effacing and eager to share the spotlight for the work, notes that uncovering the *ATG* genes in yeast was a revelation for the field of autophagy research. This made it possible for researchers to create knockout mice—lab animals who lack specific *ATG* genes—and enabled scientists to see what happens in organisms without the full complement of autophagy genes.

---

7   "Yoshinori Ohsumi Biographical." *The Nobel Prizes 2016*. Sagamore Beach: Science History Publications, a division of Watson Publishing International LLC, 2017.

It also won Yoshinori Ohsumi the Nobel Prize in Physiology or Medicine in 2016, a real turning point in the tale of autophagy. He stepped to the podium to collect his prize, taking the time to thank yeast for its contribution to his work and for the gifts of sake and liquor. This area of research, which his colleagues once considered weird, now received a staggering uptick in interest. Journals that once published only a few relevant articles each week now boomed to accommodate more than 60 articles every single week.

And Ohsumi? His work simply continues. His lab at the Tokyo Institute of Technology hopes to unravel even more of autophagy's mysteries: its products, subtle influences on metabolic pathways, and the links between genetics and disease. His original paper identifying the *ATG* genes is still the most-cited paper in the field.

BUT THE STORY BEGINS MUCH EARLIER

The first act of the lysosome story opens in the 1950s. While little Ohsumi was still scouring the natural areas around his childhood home for bugs and other artifacts, Belgian cytologist and biochemist Christian de Duve's career was redirected by his own curiosity and an unexpected laboratory observation.[8]

While investigating insulin using rat livers, de Duve noticed that the cells he was studying kicked up the release of the enzyme acid phosphatase in proportion to how damaged the cells were by a centrifuge. Cells beaten up by the spinner dumped more enzyme. This peculiarity, called enzyme latency, had absolutely no bearing on de Duve's research, but his curiosity couldn't be quashed. He followed the trail

---

8   Christian de Duve – Biographical. NobelPrize.org. Nobel Media AB 2019. March 8, 2019. https://www.nobelprize.org/prizes/medicine/1974/duve/biographical.

to discover that the cell had membrane-bound subsections, essentially intracellular sacks chock-full of the enzyme.

After viewing those same sacks (or organelles, as they say) under an electron microscope, an American biologist named Alex Novikoff confirmed them as enzymatic organelles, christened them lysosomes, and produced the first images of them. De Duve would go on to win a Nobel Prize in 1974 for his work on lysosomes, but Novikoff would not, thanks to a surge in McCarthyism that upended his career.

Novikoff—who'd joined the Communist Party as a student in the 1930s and worked for the teachers' union—refused to go before the Senate to name and shame his communist friends some 20 years later when the Red Scare rocked the US government. As a result, he was soundly dismissed from his tenured position at the University of Vermont College of Medicine. Fast forward another 30 years, and that same university would offer Novikoff an honorary degree as an apology for his mistreatment. The ship had sailed on the Nobel Prize, however, despite de Duve's insistence that Novikoff's boldness and creativity had made the lysosome's discovery possible.

There were other contributors who paved the way for Ohsumi, too, both in terms of tech and scientific discovery. The electron microscope, first built in the 1930s, made it possible for early researchers to watch the formation and fusing of the autophagosome in real time, and for two other researchers, named Arstila and Trump, to see the double membrane bubble.

And if you look back even further, the first description of phagocytosis— that Pac-Man–like engulfment of particles—dates all the way to 1882. Russian zoologist Ilya Mechnikov slid tiny thorns from his tangerine tree (who even knew citrus trees have thorns?) into starfish larvae (as one does) and watched white blood cells rush to the site as a pathogen-killing inflammatory response. He called those gobbling cells "phagocytes" and earned the 1908 Nobel Prize. Since they challenged the conventional belief that white blood cells spread infection, which was a game changer, his observations also scored him the nickname "father of natural immunity" among present-day immunologists.

In his biographical statement, Yoshinori Ohsumi took great pains to acknowledge the predecessors and colleagues who paved the way for his discoveries and participated in his research. In fact, one of the most compelling threads of the autophagy tale is the way the scientific community freely shared the work and research materials along the way. From Ohsumi running over to his colleagues' electron microscope or his wife's lab to de Duve standing up for Novikoff to research teams sharing knockout mice, there's an element of teamwork here that feels like good medicine for the particular ills of 2019.

CHAPTER 3

FUTURE RESEARCH TARGETS

LOOKING FORWARD

In the time since Yoshinori Ohsumi accepted the 2016 Nobel Prize, the field of autophagy research has seen an explosion in interest. For science journalists, enthusiasts, and researchers keeping track of the discoveries, the literature yield is now staggering. Plug the term "autophagy" into the search bar at PubMed—the search engine that queries Medline, which is maintained by the US National Library of Medicine at the National Institutes of Health—and you'll return over 2,000 pages of results containing over 40,000 highly relevant entries. In the weeks between writing this section and coming back to revise it, PubMed added almost 100 pages of entries, representing over 1,000 brand-spanking-new journal articles. To say the field is hot is an understatement.

But what exactly are those researchers investigating? A simpler (ha!) question might be: What are the current goals of autophagy research?

One target remains essentially the same as Ohsumi's objective when he set out to characterize the autophagy genome. Researchers want to unravel the secrets of the autophagy lysosomal pathway. This includes uncovering the precise mechanisms for regulating the cell program *in vivo* (within the living)—and what dysregulation looks like. This means looking at both autophagy and other cell programs (such as metabolism) that interact with the program or influence it. It also means looking at noncanonical autophagy, which are alternate pathways the cell program can take that skip some of the core machinery of regular autophagy.

Researchers also want to figure out the precise roles that autophagy plays in influencing disease outcomes and maneuver those findings into accessible treatment options. The science is no doubt interesting in its own right, but real-life people with real-life concerns about disease (either because they already have a diagnosis or have highly personal reasons to worry about one down the road) always hope that the fruit of research will be more than just interesting ideas. The people want solutions! And they want drugs! And they'd really like those things tailored to their individual needs.

TAKE TWO AND CALL ME IN THE MORNING

There is no question that autophagy is druggable. That is, there are molecular targets researchers can use to amp autophagy up or tamp it down (or block it altogether) as a disease intervention. Of course, this means looking forward to more than just new pharmaceutical commercials for yet more pills. "Druggable" is a broad descriptor that includes the development of new drugs; the repurposing of existing drugs for new applications; experimental treatment tools like gene therapy; efforts to make vaccines more effective; and techniques for preventing disease development or recurrence.

And the potential areas of influence are both vast and broad: aging, cancer, cardiovascular disease, genetic conditions, infectious disease, neurodegenerative illnesses, and even conditions like heavy metal poisoning. Just a couple of years out from Ohsumi's prize, the question is not if, but when, what, and under what conditions?

Inquiring minds specifically want to know:

- What diseases or conditions will be the first to see an autophagy drug or treatment?

   Nobody can see the future, but probably something serious enough that the benefits outweigh any risks or side effects. Some real contenders are infectious diseases or infections caused by antibiotics-resistant organisms (check out Chapter 5); diabetes, which has reached epidemic levels, according to the World Health Organization (see Chapter 6); and cancer, since it has such high stakes and research funding (Chapter 8).

- Can pharmacological agents be as effective as natural approaches for triggering autophagy?

   It's hard to say. While the natural options are part and parcel of how autophagy works and therefore most effective, a pill or drug would sure make it easier for regular people (and especially sick people) to access.

- What political factors will influence the decisions related to autophagy druggability?

   Researchers are mostly looking for new drugs, since those are more profitable than repurposing approved drugs for new uses, even though the latter might be more efficient. Some experts think they would need a public sponsor to change that. This means an individual or organization (this could be an academic institution or pharmaceutical company) helps fund and sustain research and may play a liaison role with the FDA. Or, (and this is major conjecture) perhaps an overhaul of how the health care system and biomedical research relate to one another is needed as part of sweeping systemic changes to public health management.

Science consumers interested in the natural approach—jump starting autophagy through diet, exercise, and fasting regimens—probably already recognize some of these ideas from traditional or folk medicine. And this isn't woo-woo. Scientists acknowledge that these unconventional methods are the "most efficient way" to stay "young and disease-free."[9] Here, it's not so much about "making" autophagy druggable as bringing that information to a broader audience and perhaps milking science for specific recommendations and efficacy statistics. (If this is you, Part III might be your cup of organic, ethically harvested tea.)

There are downsides to those traditional methods. Namely, they can feel difficult. There's no shame in acknowledging that maintaining a regular fasting schedule or exercise program is tough, especially for people with barriers to access, like lack of regular childcare or free time. Plus, it's inevitable that druggable will eventually translate to medication. According to experts, "there is little doubt that the economic interests linked to modern medical practice as well as the attitude of the patient/consumer will ultimately favor the oral or parenteral (injectable) use of fully synthetic compounds."[10]

---

9   Maria Chiara Maiuri and Guido Kroemer. "Therapeutic Modulation of Autophagy: Which Disease Comes First?" *Cell Death and Differentiation* 26 (2019):680–89. https://doi .org/10.1038/s41418-019-0290-0.

10   Maiuri, "Therapeutic Modulation of Autophagy," 680–89.

SO, WHAT COMES FIRST?

The open questions then are which diseases will leap to the forefront in clinical trials, and will these drugs and interventions target autophagy in general or seek to modify selective autophagy, such as specific types of cargo or pathways? Going deeper, will those interventions look at acute issues such as drug-resistant bacteria or organ failure? Or will researchers set their sights on a chronic illness or even the universal condition of aging? Some scientists speculate that the first target for clinically approved autophagy modulation will likely be a "severe, rapidly developing disease" since the stakes are higher and outweigh the potential side effects.[11]

And what of the drugs that already exist? Repurposing approved drugs for new uses is part and parcel of drug development. Researchers point to a broad selection of already-approved drugs they know to be autophagy inducers.[12] These include aspirin, ambroxol, carbamazepine, cysteamine, rilmenidine, and valproic acid. Since these are already approved for other uses and have established toxicology profiles, researchers could theoretically skip the first phase of clinical trials and speed up the timeline of their approval for a new use.

However, some researchers think this scenario is unlikely. The reason? It's just more lucrative to bring a hot new drug to the market than to repurpose an established drug. According to those researchers, only a public sponsor backing clinical evaluation of existing autophagy inducers would make this seemingly obvious step probable.

Either way, scientists need pharmacokinetic data that traces what happens to a substance from the moment it enters the human body, and target-engagement biomarkers for autophagy modulators to help

---

11 Maiuri, "Therapeutic Modulation of Autophagy," 680–89.

12 Maiuri, 680–89.

figure out proper dosing and make sure that the results of clinical trials truly reflect what's going on.[13]

PERSONALIZED CARE: THE FUTURE OF MEDICINE?

It's hard to discuss autophagy research and the likelihood of clinical autophagy modulators without also talking about the changing landscape of medicine. Emerging scientific fields and technologies, especially the -omics disciplines (which explore genes, proteins, and low-molecular-weight compounds) and next-generation gene sequencing, promise a real shift in the way people think about health care and what they expect from clinicians.

Where medical decisions once focused on pathology and trial and error, the shifting landscape in medicine now encourages gathering sophisticated, highly personal data to tailor treatment to the specific patient. One physician researcher uses pancreatitis as a model for how personalized medicine works.[14] The old medical model assumed that pancreatitis almost always resulted from heavy drinking, end of story. But newer technologies revealed this is only a small portion of cases (about 15 percent in the study), with more significant percentages of cases triggered by unknown causes (42 percent) and genetics (24 percent). In fact, the disease has a single molecular cause—trypsinogen activation—but the triggers that underlie it are quite varied.

For this reason, health-care providers using a personalized approach would group patients based on behavioral risk factors and genetic

13 Steven Finkbeiner. "The Autophagy Lysosomal Pathway and Neurodegeneration," *Cold Spring Harbor Perspectives in Biology* (2019). https://doi.org/10.1101/cshperspect .a033993.

14 David C. Whitcomb. "What Is Personalized Medicine and What Should It Replace?" *National Reviews in Gastroenterology and Hepatology* 9, no. 7 (2012): 418–24. https://doi. org/10.1038/nrgastro.2012.100.

biomarkers for treatment planning. After all, patients with genetic mutations that affect the structure and function of the pancreas need different treatment than patients who develop pancreatitis for a non-genetic reason, such as an obstruction or an underlying autoimmune problem.

When it comes to tapping into a major cell program like autophagy and leveraging it into treatment options (in other words, making it druggable), it makes sense to imagine this in the context of personal-ized medicine, even if many or most patients are still stuck with health care from the old paradigm. The complex relationships among cell programs, the vast numbers of genes implicated in these processes, and even the complicated way autophagy plays out in some diseases (especially cancer) all point toward complex webs of information rather than discrete yes/no, up/down cures.

All these things, from the explosion of autophagy research and the striking numbers of diseases and conditions mediated by autophagy to the push for personalized medicine and even the possibility of systemic changes to health care on the horizon (or not, who knows?), could come together with autophagy-based treatments acting as a bridge from the current medical model to a personalized one.

In his Nobel Prize banquet speech, Yoshinori Ohsumi describes life as "a delicate balance between continuous synthesis and degradation."[15] For biologists, that breaking down is just as important as the build-ing up. Ohsumi also noted how good it feels to see the explosion of research in his field and to imagine his contributions playing a trans-forming role in conquering human disease. It's tempting to read those words and also imagine the potential for autophagy to tear down and rebuild an expiring medical model.

---

15 "Yoshinori Ohsumi Banquet Speech." *The Nobel Prizes 2016.* https://www.nobelprize
.org/prizes/medicine/2016/ohsumi/25025-yoshinori-ohsumi-banquet-speech-2016.

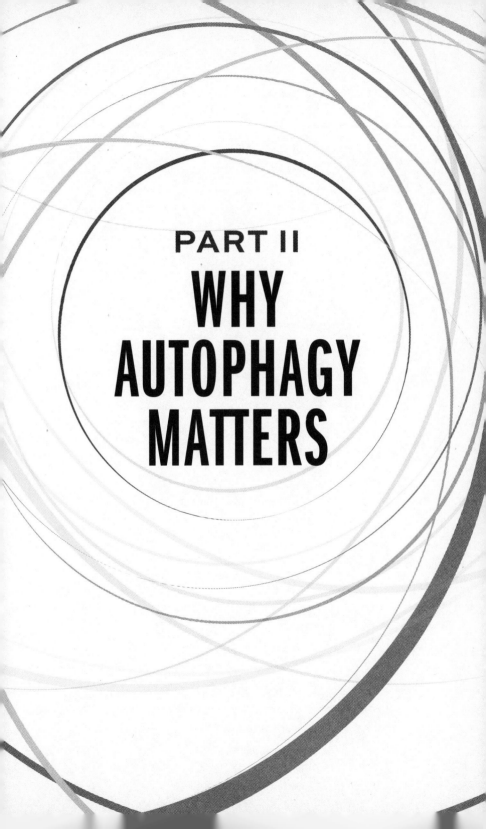

PART II
WHY AUTOPHAGY MATTERS

CHAPTER 4

LONGEVITY

FOREVER YOUNG

Mortality is the (hungry) wolf at the door. And humans, in true human form, have tried to evade its grasp basically forever. The earliest and best-known reference to the quest for immortality is probably the fountain of youth. Around the 5th century BCE, the ancient Greek historian Herodotus described a pool of water in which the Macrobians—mythical people from either the horn of Africa or India, depending on whom you read—bathed. The water was oily and smelled of violets and anything you dropped into it sank to the bottom, no matter how light. Dunking regularly in the fountain preserved the Macrobians well and enabled them to live into their 120s. Things got really classy when they did kick the bucket, because they practiced an elaborate embalming ritual: propping up the restored cadaver inside a crystal pillar in the home for about a year. The Macrobians were a lot of things: tall, wealthy (they even chained up their prisoners with gold), easy on the eyes, creative with their dead...and enviously long-lived.

That desire to find a magic fountain and, with it, eternal youth seems silly on its face, but is it really that different from what scientists hope to do? If you search PubMed again, this time for research aimed at halting or reversing normal aging, the results run the gamut from rad to revolting. Have you heard of heterochronic parabiosis?[16] It means "living beside," and it entails taking two separate animals—usually an old/young pair of lab mice—and stitching them together so they share a bloodstream. This literally pumps the young mouse's blood through the body of the older mouse and yields benefits like improving the life span of the older mouse and reversing brain changes in a murine Alzheimer's model. It's a method best summed up with a shuddery WTF (corpses in crystal pillars don't seem so weird now, huh?) and also happens to be the way researchers gained life-preserving insight into the endocrine and immune systems. Taking this from animal models to human studies—meaning transfusing the blood or plasma of young donors into older people—is a legitimate research interest. (It's also the bipartisan platform of the 2020 presidential election.)

Whether you hope to bathe in a literal fountain of youth, hook up your aging self to a spry plasma donor, or spend your time slathering on age-defying lotions and eating superfoods, the dream of beating old age is real. Mark Twain said it like this: "Life would be infinitely happier if we could only be born at the age of 80 and gradually approach 18."[17]

ENTER THE AUTOPHAGY LAB

Increasing the human life span is probably the most-cited aspect of autophagy research. The autophagy cell program is so unequivocally linked with longevity that scientists believe amping up the expression

---

16   Shetty, "Emerging Anti-Aging Strategies—Scientific Basis and Efficacy," 1165–84.

17   Willie Drye. "Fountain of Youth," *National Geographic*. Accessed January 16, 2019. https://www.nationalgeographic.com/archaeology-and-history/archaeology/fountain-of-youth/.

of *ATG* genes is actually a "prerequisite for life span extension."[18] The opposite holds true, too: Dropping autophagy levels in young animals makes them age prematurely.[19] You simply can't have a long life without a strong autophagy program.

Scientists have known for about a century that restricting the calories available to lab animals slows down their aging and extends their lives.[20] This holds true in labs working with mice, worms, flies, yeast, fish, dogs, and apes. Some scientists say calorie restriction is the "most consistently reproducible experimental means of...extending average and maximum life span in model organisms of aging."[21] Figuring out why this worked took longer. And—surprise!— it was autophagy.

The first evidence that the life span–extending mechanism was actually the autophagy lysosomal pathway came from studies with the simple, millimeter-long worm *Caenorhabditis elegans*. Scientists found that when they knocked down the *ATG* genes of these nematode friends, suppressing the expression of certain genes that drive autophagy, they produced worms with shorter lives who also appeared old by measures, such as reduced motility. Just like old humans, prematurely aged worms had a harder time getting around.[22]

18   Frank Madeo et al. "Essential Role for Autophagy in Life Span Extension," *Journal of Clinical Investigation* 125, no. 1 (2015):85–93. https://doi.org/10.1172/JCI73946.

19   Shuhei Nakamura and Tamotsu Yoshimori. "Autophagy and Longevity," *Molecules and Cells* 41, no. 1 (2018):65–72. https://doi.org/10.14348/molcells.2018.2333.

20   Shuhei Nakamura et al., 65–72.

21   Bradley J. Willcox and Donald Craig Willcox. "Caloric Restriction, CR Mimetics, and Healthy Aging in Okinawa: Controversies and Clinical Implications," *Current Opinions in Clinical Nutrition and Metabolic Care* 17, no. 1 (2014):51–58. https://doi.org/10.1097/MC.00000000000000019.

22   Sara Gelino et al. "Intestinal Autophagy Improves Healthspan and Longevity in C. Elegans during Dietary Restriction," *PLOS Genetics* 12, no. 7 (2017):e1006135. https://doi.org/10.1371/journal.pgen.1006135.

Drosophila fruit flies showed a similar pattern with reductions in both life span and climbing activity among knockdown flies.[23] Lab mice with autophagy inhibited in their skeletal muscle cells also have reductions in life span, body strength, and synaptic function in their brains.[24]

When scientists trigger autophagy using calorie restriction or compounds that enhance autophagy, they see the opposite pattern. Lab rats on restricted diets live almost twice as long as their peers, and they showed improvements to heart rate and blood pressure within one week.[25] This holds true for primates, too. Lab monkeys and humans both show extended life spans with calorie restriction intended to upregulate autophagy. Mice treated with autophagy enhancers (like spermidine) also had longer lives, and scientists who perform observational epidemiology note reductions in mortality rates among humans who enjoyed spermidine-rich diets, too.[26]

The overall pattern is this: Autophagy levels naturally decrease with age, opening the door for cell changes associated with age-related disease and mortality, like the accumulation of DNA mutation damage as well as clumping proteins. However, kicking up the expression of autophagy genes "protects from aging," removing those problematic cell changes and stretching the life span.[27]

---

23 Gelino, "Intestinal Autophagy Improves Healthspan and Longevity in C. Elegans during Dietary Restriction."

24 Gelino, "Intestinal Autophagy Improves Healthspan and Longevity in C. Elegans during Dietary Restriction."

25 Mark P Mattson et al. "Impact of Intermittent Fasting on Health and Disease Processes," *Ageing Research Review* 39 (2017):46–58. https://doi.org/10.1016/j.arr.2016.10.005.

26 Maiuri, "Therapeutic Modulation of Autophagy: Which Disease Comes First?" 680–89.

27 Aurelian Udristioiu and Delia Nica-Badea. "Autophagy Dysfunctions Associated with Cancer Cells and Their Therapeutic Implications," *Biomedicine & Pharmacotherapy* 115 (2019): 108892. https://doi.org/10.1016/j.biopha.2019.108892.

LIKE A FINE F-ING WINE

Of course, longevity is about more than just living as long as you possibly can. Quality of life—called health span among researchers—is a better measure of success for human subjects. What's the point of living forever if you can't enjoy it?

The tension between longer lives and age-related conditions is at an all-time high. Life expectancy has almost doubled in the past century, and it's not stopping there. Scientists expect the over-65 sector to climb to about 25 percent of the US population by 2060 (which is, ahem, elder millennials), and this brings an increase in age-related diseases.[28] Some researchers pragmatically describe aging as "the functional deterioration of an organism"; you get older, and stuff starts to break down.[29]

Researchers define "successful aging" as older adults (in their 60s to 80s) with no significant disease or age-related disability, reasonable cognitive function, and the ability to lead active lives.[30] Defying the usual changes that come with age is downright revolutionary. One scientist describes prolonging the health span as "subverting" the cause of age-related disorders rather than simply looking for stop-gap treatments to deal with the symptoms.[31]

Valter Longo, whose work features prominently in this book and who created an eating-and-fasting plan for the express purpose of extending the human health span, doesn't even call what he studies aging, preferring the term juventology.[32] This is more than just a simple turn of phrase. Moving from a research paradigm that looks at aging (you

---

28 Shetty, "Emerging Anti-aging Strategies—Scientific Basis and Efficacy," *Aging and Disease* 9, no. 6 (2018):1165–84. https://doi.org/10.14336/AD.2018.1026.

29 Nakamura, "Autophagy and Longevity," 65–72.

30 Shetty, "Emerging Anti-aging Strategies—Scientific Basis and Efficacy, 1165–84.

31 Madeo, "Essential Role for Autophagy in Life Span Extension," 85–93.

32 Valter Longo. *The Longevity Diet*. New York: Avery, Penguin Group, 2018.

know, that pesky functional deterioration) to one that focuses on maintaining youthfulness even as the years add up shifts the conversation about longevity.

When it comes to subverting age-related disease and aging successfully, researchers believe amping up autophagy through whole-organism methods like fasting or using autophagy-enhancing supplements can extend the human life span and delay onset of age-related diseases.[33] These include the conditions outlined in the next chapters: infectious disease, immune problems, metabolic disorders, neurodegenerative diseases, and cancers.[34]

It also includes one of the most readily obvious measures of aging: your skin. Researchers are just beginning to investigate the role autophagy might play in skin health, particularly as it relates to aging. They know that the cell program amps up in skin cells after exposure to the coarse particulate matter present in air pollution, which can cause skin inflammation and signs of aging, such as pigment spots, deep wrinkles, and impaired collagen synthesis. It likely also plays a role in skin cancer and both inflammatory and infectious skin diseases. Early evidence suggests that autophagy may be reparative under all those circumstances.[35] Researchers have already linked autophagy with treating skin damage from UV exposure, skin fragility (which may arise with autophagy impairment), psoriasis, allergic contact dermatitis, and

33   Guido Kroemer. "Autophagy: A Druggable Process That Is Deregulated in Aging and Human Disease," *Journal of Clinical Investigation* 125, no. 1 (2015):1–4. https://doi.org/10.1172/JCI78652.

34   Shetty, "Emerging Anti-aging Strategies—Scientific Basis and Efficacy," 1165–84.

35   Park, Seo-Yeon et al. "Air Pollution, Autophagy, and Skin Aging: Impact of Particulate Matter (PM_{10}) on Human Dermal Fibroblasts." *International Journal of Molecular Sciences* 19, no. 9 (2018): 2727. https://doi.org/10.3390/ijms19092727.

both squamous cell carcinoma, a common form of skin cancer, and melanoma.[36, 37]

However, it's not totally clear precisely how autophagy and skin cells interact. Some early research suggests that the relationship is much more complex than autophagy simply declining as you age. In fact, some signs of aging probably show up because the damage has accumulated to the point that the normal autophagy program simply can't keep up.[38] Regardless, there's good reason to believe that novel therapies for serious skin conditions and the effects of normal aging on your skin may be on the horizon as skin-specific research into autophagy modulation grows. To make that happen, researchers say they need a standardized method for monitoring changes in autophagy over time.

The link between calorie restriction (CR) and longevity is so compelling that the US National Institute on Aging has declared it a priority research focus. When scientists want to look at longevity, they often turn to the decades of data compiled about traditional Okinawans.[39] This population is the only known group with an extended maximum life span, boasting five times the number of centenarians compared with other industrialized populations. Using a measure for life expectancy past 65, researchers know that elderly Americans can expect to live until 81 or 84, depending on sex assignment, while elderly Okinawans can expect to live until 83 or 89. That's an extra couple of years for men, but half a decade more for women. When it comes

36   Y. Wang et al. "Insights into Autophagy Machinery in Cells Related to Skin Diseases and Strategies for Therapeutic Modulation." *Biomedicine & Pharmacotherapy* 113 (2019): 108775. https://doi.org/10.1016/j.biopha.2019.108775.

37   Y. Guo et al. "Autophagy in Skin Diseases." *Dermatology* 235, no. 5 (2019): 380–89. https://doi.org/10.1159/000500470.

38   Hei Sung Kim et al. "Autophagy in Human Skin Fibroblasts: Impact of Age." *International Journal of Molecular Sciences* 19, no. 8 (2018): 2254. https://doi.org/10.3390/ijms19082254.

39   Willcox, "Caloric Restriction, CR Mimetics, and Healthy Aging in Okinawa: Controversies and Clinical Implications," 51–58.

to health span, the stats are similarly skewed positive for Okinawans. They have much lower rates of age-related conditions like cardiovascular disease, cancer, and dementia.

The likely reason behind this—and the reason researchers look at traditional Okinawan data to better understand CR—is that those healthy 100-year-olds consumed approximately 40 percent fewer calories than the average adult in the US. Some of the most startling evidence that traditional Okinawan longevity correlates with CR (and not just good genes or something) is that younger Okinawans who don't follow the traditional CR diet don't see the advantages their elders do. In fact, their stats are slightly worse than those for mainland Japanese or American people.

According to scientists using the Okinawa data, the anti-aging benefits of CR are most robust until reaching about half the typical calorie intake, and when performed in a way that ensures no nutritional deficiencies.[40] The autophagy-related mechanisms for traditional Okinawans aren't just very-low-calorie diets, either. The data suggests that many of the staple foods for the population are CR mimetics, compounds that provide the benefits of CR even in the absence of food restriction. These include phytochemicals found in sweet potatoes, marine foods, turmeric, and soy-based flavonoids. And scientists speculate that foods local to Okinawa are naturally rich in these phytochemicals because those compounds exist to protect the plant from cellular stress (think: extra-powerful UV light) specific to the island's location.

---

40 Willcox, 51–58.

THE TAKEAWAY

Your body relies on the autophagy lysosomal pathway to keep mortality and age-related diseases at bay. There is good evidence fasting or calorie restriction is the single most powerful DIY tool at your disposal for ensuring that your autophagy program runs smoothly for as many years as possible, stacking the odds for a long, healthy stretch of old age. The ideal time frame for adopting a fasting regimen is middle age, commencing sometime in the late 30s or early 40s. It isn't generally considered safe to fast without supervision after age 65 or if you have health conditions that require monitoring by a health-care provider.

CHAPTER 5

IMMUNE SYSTEM AND CHRONIC ILLNESS

DEFENSE AGAINST INVADERS

While a major function of the autophagy lysosomal pathway is cleaning up old organelles and misfolded proteins, that's not all it does. Autophagy also plays a primary role in immune response. Your cells use autophagy as an "effector arm of the immune system" to round up and destroy the pathogens invading your cells in order to keep you healthy.[41]

Your immune system includes innate and adaptive responses. Innate immunity is your immune system's first line of defense. It's quick and evolutionarily old, but it has downsides. It's not terribly sensitive to fine distinctions among pathogens, and it's not the most powerful option. Your innate immune system also doesn't learn from its encounters with germs.

---

41   Daniel Puleston and Anna Katharina Simon. "Autophagy in the Immune System," *Immunology* 141, no. 1 (2014): 1–8. https://doi.org/10.1111/imm.12165.

Your adaptive immunity, on the other hand, is a newer adaptation that mounts more slowly but recognizes subtle differences among pathogens and responds with more oomph. It also learns from its experiences with germs, so the second or third time your adaptive immunity runs into a specific pathogen, it can respond more efficiently. This is why you can mount a quicker, more robust response to disease-causing microbes after having the illness or receiving a vaccine.

The type of autophagy that clears harmful pathogens—xenophagy— is almost certainly the earliest form of innate immune response.[42] To make it work, the immune system uses pattern recognition receptors to find pathogenic microbes (think: intracellular bacteria or viruses) that seem foreign to the cell. Then, it triggers the autophagy program to eliminate those invaders before they can harm you. The xenophagy path simply forms a double-membraned autophagosome, engulfs the pathogen, and carries it off for destruction. An alternate pathway, LC3-associated phagocytosis (LAP), is also autophagy-related but much more complex.

Scientists know that this primitive immune function is related to autophagy because defects in *ATG* genes predispose carriers to infectious disease. They have also established that stimulating xenophagy can help patients with cystic fibrosis clear the opportunistic bacteria *Pseudomonas aeruginosa* and help other patients fight off the TB-causing bacteria *Mycobacterium tuberculosis*. These findings even suggest that autophagy may be key for dealing with antibiotic-resistant infections.[43]

Autophagy plays a role in adaptive immunity, too. It ensures the survival of specialized white blood cells called T cells, which are the major boots-on-the-ground soldiers of the adaptive immune response. And

---

42   Maiuri, "Therapeutic Modulation of Autophagy: Which Disease Comes First?" 680–89.
43   Maiuri, 680–89.

it aids in the formation of memory CD8+ T cells, which "remember" those previous infections or vaccines.

A WORMY SITUATION

Researchers think autophagy's immunosurveillance role makes it a promising model for developing new drugs to combat parasites.[44] The bulk of parasitic infections show up in the most marginalized communities within low-income nations, but not always. The Centers for Diseases Control (CDC) has targeted one class of these—the neglected parasitic infections (NPIs)—as a public health priority.[45]

These NPIs include:

- **Chagas**. Caused by the bloodsucking kissing bug *Trypanosoma cruzi;* affects over 8 million people in Latin America alone with symptoms like fever and abdominal pain

- **Cysticercosis**. Causes seizures, thanks to the larval cysts of the tapeworm *Taenia solium*; often transmitted in low-income areas with free-ranging pigs

- **Toxocariasis**. Comes from roundworms *Toxocara canis* and *Toxocara cati*, found in household dogs and cats and usually ingested with contaminated dirt; symptoms depend on affected organs and can include fever, fatigue, breathing problems, and visual impairment

---

44 Henryka Dlugonska. "Autophagy as a Universal Intracellular Process. A Comment on the 2016 Nobel Prize in Physiology or Medicine," *Annals of Parasitology* 63, no. 3 (2017): 153–57. https://doi.org/10.17420/ap6303.100.

45 Centers for Disease Control. "Parasites—Neglected Parasitic Infections." 2018 https://www.cdc.gov/parasites/npi.

- **Toxoplasmosis**. A foodborne illness affecting over 40 million people in the United States, many of whom are unwitting carriers since a robust immune system keeps the parasite in check. Notably the leading cause of foodborne illness–related deaths, marked by fever, fatigue, headache, and muscle aches

- **Trichomoniasis**. A sexually transmitted infection by *Trichomonas vaginalis* that is asymptomatic for 70 percent of people (or may bring abdominal pain and genital discomfort) and increases the likelihood of infection by other STIs, including HIV

Okay, that's ruined your appetite, but how likely are you to encounter an NPI or other parasitic infection, assuming you live somewhere industrialized, have boring travel and eating habits, and always follow safety guidelines for pet care and food prep? Actually…more likely than you might think.

This is especially true as climate change blurs the artificial economic boundaries between humans. New patterns of human migration and rising sea levels could usher parasites into unexpected places. And scientists estimate that climate change may wipe out as many as one-third of all parasites, which doesn't work out in humans' favor, since these extinction events will probably include "unpredictable invasions" and general bioinstability for their hosts (spoiler: that's you).[46]

This is why researchers who work with parasites want to figure out the mechanisms that control the interactions between these parasitic infections and the autophagy cell program. They already know that triggering autophagy in mice infected with chikungunya or West Nile virus is enough to keep those rodents alive.[47] The ability to up- or

---

46   Damian Carrington. "Climate Change Could Wipe Out a Third of Parasite Species, Study Finds," *The Guardian*, September 6, 2017. https://www.theguardian.com/environment/2017/sep/06/climate-change-could-wipe-out-a-third-of-parasite-species-study-finds.

47   Maiuri, "Therapeutic Modulation of Autophagy: Which Disease Comes First?" 680–89.

down-regulate autophagy—or the expression of *ATG* genes—could change the game for people who become unwilling hosts to creepy crawlies.

PUTTING THE INFLAMMATION IN INFLAMMATORY

The other major area of immune-related autophagy research is chronic inflammatory disease. The main foot soldiers of the immune system are specialized white blood cells, including macrophages, neutrophils, and T cells. Like good soldiers, these cells follow orders letting them know where they are needed and advising them to stand down when the mission is over. Your immune cells use cell signaling molecules—inflammation factors like cytokines and chemokines—to pass those messages. These can be pro-inflammatory markers, which amp up the signal and therefore the symptoms of inflammation, or anti-inflammatory markers, which send the signal to chill and ease the symptoms of inflammation.

This coordinated response works well when dealing with acute problems like invading viruses or bacteria. Consider this: The handles of 71 percent of gas pumps and 68 percent of mailboxes are highly contaminated with germs—enough to make you sick.[48] And the faucets and door handles in airplane bathrooms? They're smeared with traces of the intestinal bacteria *Escherichia coli* 100 percent of the time. The phone in your back pocket? Ten times germier than a toilet seat—so much so that one unfortunate dude contracted Ebola after stealing

---

48   Live Science. "Germs Really Are Everywhere [infographic]," *Live Science* website. October 31, 2011. https://www.livescience.com/16787-germs-everyday-surfaces-infographic .html.

one from a quarantined area.[49] Yet people with strong immune systems don't get sick nearly as often as you might expect once you realize how gross the world is.

On the flip side, the immune system is prone to dysregulation, especially as a result of aging or illness. When that happens, it may trigger inflammation factors when it shouldn't, or low levels of inflammation can hang out and never return to the baseline. Some people's immune systems even mount robust immune responses against perfectly normal cells or cell components. This is the molecular basis of autoimmune conditions that affect about 9 percent of people (and climbing), such as inflammatory Crohn's disease, systemic lupus erythematosus (SLE), multiple sclerosis, psoriasis, rheumatoid arthritis, and type 2 diabetes.[50]

AUTOPHAGY'S COMPLICATED ROLE IN AUTOIMMUNE DISEASE

Unfortunately, while dysregulated autophagy definitely plays a role in autoimmune disease, the underlying mechanisms are unclear or even confusing. For conditions like inflammatory bowel disease and lupus, the source is likely genetic. People with common *ATG* gene variations, called polymorphisms, are predisposed to these "tissue-destructive inflammatory diseases."[51] The underlying causes of other autoimmune illnesses like multiple sclerosis and rheumatoid arthritis are less certain but probably have something to do with the way autophagy aids in

---

49   Susan E. Matthews. "Why Your Cell Phone Has More Bacteria Than a Toilet Seat," *Live Science*. August 30, 2012. https://www.livescience.com/22822-cell-phones-germs.html.

50   Sanguine Byun et al. "Therapeutic Implications of Autophagy Inducers in Immunological Disorders, Infection, and Cancer," *International Journal of Molecular Sciences* 18 (2017): 1959–81. https://doi.org/10.3390/ijms18091959.

51   Zhen Yang et al. "Autophagy in Autoimmune Disease," *Journal of Molecular Medicine (Berlin, Germany)* 93, no. 7 (2015): 707–17. https://doi.org/10.1007/s00109-015-1297-8.

the "long-term survival of adaptive immune cells,"[52] which can mistakenly attack the body's own cells or tissues with some diseases. In these cases, clinicians may try to suppress the immune system in order to protect against damage.

Scientists think that autophagy acts as a critical counterbalance to the processes the immune system uses to do its job, like inflammation. What's trickier is that some features of autoimmune diseases seem to fall on one side of that balance, while others are the opposite. This makes it more complex than "hit it with more autophagy!" In fact, since the problem is dysregulation itself, autophagy-gone-wild is just as likely to be a problem in autoimmune disease as sluggish autophagy.

To deal with this complexity, researchers hoping to discover new treatments to augment the current protocol of immunosuppressive therapy are looking for both "autophagy-inducing and autophagy-suppressing pharmacologic interventions" for folks with chronic autoimmune conditions.[53]

FASTING (OR FMD) WITH SPECIFIC AUTOIMMUNE DISEASES

MULTIPLE SCLEROSIS

The symptoms of this autoimmune disease—pain, visual impairment or loss, limb weakness, and issues with balance or muscle control—happen because the body's immune cells mistakenly attack the myelin covering that protects the nerve fibers of the central nervous system.

---

52 Yang, "Autophagy in Autoimmune Disease," 707–17.

53 Yang, 707–17.

In experiments with mice, fasting has been shown to remove old or malfunctioning immune cells while increasing the number of available stem cells. Once feeding resumes, those stem cells differentiate into immune cells, replacing the ones killed off during the fast. At the same time, progenitor cells, which behave like stem cells but with a more limited range for the kinds of cells they can become, can rebuild damaged nerves.[54]

Scientists interested in fast-mimicking diets (FMDs) have conducted human trials consisting of a seven-day FMD wherein the participants with MS consumed only 200 to 350 calories of broth and juice per day followed by six months of either a plant-based or a ketogenic diet. Participants self-reported improvements, and relapses were slightly higher in the control group, leading the study authors to plan a larger, multiple-cycle study.[55]

RHEUMATOID ARTHRITIS

This chronic autoimmune condition also results from immune cells attacking the body, producing chronic inflammation, joint pain and stiffness, and fatigue. Studies suggest that long fasts of one to three weeks in length—or very-low-calorie FMDs—improve symptoms of RA during the fasting period. Some of these improvements remain only if participants stick with a vegetarian diet after the fast.[56]

CROHN'S DISEASE AND COLITIS

Chronic inflammation of the digestive tract, or inflammatory bowel disease (IBD)—also called colitis if localized to the large intestine and Crohn's disease when it shows up anywhere else in the digestive tract—brings exhaustion, weight loss, abdominal discomfort, diarrhea

---

54 Longo, *The Longevity Diet*.
55 Longo, *The Longevity Diet*.
56 Longo, *The Longevity Diet*.

and/or constipation, rectal bleeding, and inflammation that can extend to the eyes, joints, and mouth.

Researchers recently looked at the effects of both a four-day FMD and water-only fast on a mouse model of IBD. Both protocols reduced inflammation and increased the numbers of regenerative stem cells. The FMD-treated mice also saw positive changes in their protective gut microbiota and reversed the pathology of the disease. A separate clinical trial showed a reduction in markers for systemic inflammation after three cycles of FMD.[57] The researchers speculate that the plant-derived ingredients in the supplements included in the FMD helped support the regeneration of beneficial gut bacteria.

THE TAKEAWAY

Autophagy plays an important role in the normal function of your immune system to recognize invading pathogens and round them up. If your immune system becomes dysregulated, as with age, it may become confused, targeting your own cells for elimination. The key for most biological systems is balance, and this is extra true for auto-immune conditions where hyped-up autophagy is just as problematic as sluggish autophagy. Modulating autophagy (either enhancing or suppressing) holds great possibilities for treatments—including fasting—aimed at infection, inflammatory disease, and other issues mediated by the immune system.[58]

If you have a diagnosed autoimmune disease or suspect you do, your best bet is to get together with your health-care provider and make

57   P. Rangan et al. "Fasting-Mimicking Diet Modulates Microbiota and Promotes Intestinal Regeneration to Reduce Inflammatory Bowel Disease Pathology," *Cell Reports* 26, no. 10 (2019): 2704–19. https://doi.org/10.1016/j.celrep.2019.02.019.

58   Byun, "Therapeutic Implications of Autophagy Inducers in Immunological Disorders, Infection, and Cancer," 1959–81.

a solid plan together. Talk to your provider about the possibility of joining ongoing clinical trials if you want to try some of the protocols described here.

CHAPTER 6

METABOLIC CONDITIONS

NOT SO SWEET

Your pancreas contains millions of bunches of cells collectively called islets of Langerhans. Some of these cells—your beta cells—monitor the blood for circulating glucose and produce the hormone insulin in response. This signaling molecule has an important role: to bind with target cells, such as muscle cells, and tell them to take in glucose for energy. Insulin resistance, which occurs as a result of metabolic disorders and also as a side effect of aging, is when your cells stop responding well to insulin, which makes it difficult for glucose to enter your cells.

With type 1 diabetes (once called juvenile diabetes or insulin-dependent diabetes), the immune system destroys the insulin-producing beta cells. The underlying cause for this attack might be genetic, virus-mediated, a result of exposure to environmental toxins or circumstances (including trauma), or some combination of those. With type

2 diabetes (once called adult-onset diabetes or non-insulin dependent diabetes), the pancreas still produces insulin, but it isn't enough—or the target cells don't receive the insulin signal effectively.

The incidence of diagnosed diabetes has increased starkly; the US prevalence rate was just under 1 percent in 1958 but clocked in at over 7 percent in 2015. This means 1.6 million people had a diabetes diagnosis in 1958 compared with 23.4 million people with that diagnosis in 2015. And this upward trend holds true around the globe.[59] That's pretty staggering, but check this: Diabetes is responsible for more deaths each year than breast cancer and AIDS combined. It's the seventh leading cause of death in the US. And having diabetes means your chances of heart attack are double. It's also fair to say that diabetes is an age-related condition; just over 25 percent of Americans over 65 have diabetes.[60]

The economic cost of diabetes is equally shocking. The total annual expenditure associated with diagnosed diabetes in the US—and that doesn't include people who don't know they have the disease, which adds another 7.2 million people to the earlier figure—comes in at $327 billion. Every. Year. The average person with diabetes spends more than double on medical costs compared to someone without the disease.[61]

59 Centers for Disease Control. "Long-Term Trends in Diabetes," April 2017. https://www .cdc.gov/diabetes/statistics/slides/long_term_trends.pdf.

60 American Diabetes Association. "Statistics about Diabetes," American Diabetes Association website. March 22, 2018. http://www.diabetes.org/diabetes-basics/statistics/ ?loc=db-slabnav.

61 American Diabetes Association, "Statistics about Diabetes."

AUTOPHAGY TO THE RESCUE

In the flurry of research interest in the autophagy lysosomal pathway, the potential link between the cell program and metabolic conditions like diabetes seemed obvious: "Autophagy deficiency due to aging, genetic causes, or other factors could compromise an organism's ability to adapt to metabolic stress and predispose it to the development of metabolic syndrome and diabetes."[62]

This is logical since autophagy is a conserved response to metabolic stress, like the depletion of nutrients or oxygen. When those dip too low and the cell senses it's starving or stressed, it kicks up the autophagy program to break down unnecessary cell components it can use for energy. Given that direct association with metabolism, it's no surprise that disordered metabolism—diabetes, insulin resistance, and metabolic syndrome—can show up with dysregulated autophagy.

As with most research related to human disease, scientists turned to mouse models to explore diabetes. Lab mice are good choices for most animal studies, and animal studies confirmed that deficient autophagy stacks the cards against flexibly responding to metabolic stress and plays a role in the development of diabetes. However, mice aren't a perfect model for all human systems or diseases, and murine models for diabetes break down a bit because of species-specific differences in proteins called islet amyloid polypeptides (IAPP).

These proteins are amyloidogenic, or prone to clump together, in humans. This is good news for humans with diabetes, since autophagy preferentially clears protein clumps or tangles, including human IAPP clumps. Thanks to this evolutionary development (amyloidogenicity),

---

62   J. Kim et al. "The Role of Autophagy in Systemic Metabolism and Human-Type Diabetes," *Molecules and Cells* 41, no. 1 (2018): 11–17. https://doi.org/10.14348/molcells.2018.2228.

any benefit conveyed by amping up autophagy in mouse models of diabetes is much more likely to help out humans with the disease. Researchers think this makes autophagy enhancement a good strategy for dealing with the spike in metabolic syndrome and diabetes around the globe.[63]

UPPING THE PROGRAM

It's also logical that triggering autophagy using the most efficient natural method—fasting—is tricky for people with diabetes, since this condition usually requires tight regulation of eating, blood sugar checks, and insulin therapy. Fasting and fast-mimicking diets can be downright dangerous for people who manage diabetes using injected insulin. When people with diabetes inject insulin, the hormone produces a drop in glucose levels, and injecting insulin while fasting or near-fasting can drop glucose levels so quickly and steeply that it produces hypoglycemic shock and even death. This is solid "don't try this at home" territory.

That said, autophagy enhancement using cycles of FMD has been shown to reverse the symptoms of diabetes in mice and even regenerate healthy beta cells capable of producing insulin.[64] The latter actually turned on pancreatic genes usually only activated *in utero*—almost like a pancreas reset. Other researchers hope that CR mimetics might open a door for the development of autophagy-enhancing medications that could be prescribed as part of standard diabetes treatment.

63   J. Kim, "The Role of Autophagy in Systemic Metabolism and Human-Type Diabetes," 11–17.

64   Longo, *The Longevity Diet.*

CARDIOVASCULAR DISEASE AND OTHER COMORBIDITIES

One of the concerning aspects of diabetes is that it increases the risk for developing other conditions, or comorbidities that occur along with a primary condition, including cardiovascular diseases. This possibility points to one of the sure benefits of autophagy: its protective function for the cardiovascular system. According to one scientist author, "accumulating evidence suggests that repeated or continuous autophagy stimulation can protect against most if not all signs of cardiovascular aging including arteriosclerosis, increased arterial stiffness, and cardiac failure. For this reason, dietary and pharmacological measures for enhancing autophagy might be considered for the prevention of cardiovascular diseases, perhaps in the context of a general strategy to promote healthy aging."[65] It seems logical that for people who are at increased risk for developing cardiovascular disease, as is the case for people who have diabetes, the protective function of autophagy against cardiovascular problems would be even more relevant.

Having diabetes also increases the risk of developing dementia, especially Alzheimer's disease or vascular dementia, which is damage that occurs as a result of decreased blood flow in the brain. The Mayo Clinic says that many people with diabetes show the brain changes characteristic of Alzheimer's and vascular dementia in a short time frame, and that the metabolic and neurodegenerative conditions seem to work to make each other worse over time.[66] The specific link between diabetes and Alzheimer's disease is so profound that some people have proposed calling diabetes-associated Alzheimer's disease "type 3 diabetes."

---

65   Maiuri, "Therapeutic Modulation of Autophagy: Which Disease Comes First?" 680–89.

66   Mayo Clinic. "Diabetes and Alzheimer's Linked," April 19, 2019. https://www.mayo clinic.org/diseases-conditions/alzheimers-disease/in-depth/diabetes-and-alzheimers/ART-20046987.

THE TAKEAWAY

Dysregulated autophagy makes it difficult for the body to mount a flexible, robust response to metabolic stress, and predisposes those people to conditions like diabetes. The human and economic costs associated with diabetes are very high, and incidence is climbing, especially among people over 65. The development of diabetes ultimately puts people at risk for comorbid disorders, such as cardiovascular disease and dementia. Enhancing autophagy produces marked results, including regenerating the damaged beta cells that are a hallmark of diabetes. However, fasting and FMDs can be very dangerous for people who use injected insulin to control diabetes and may even be a deadly combination. Never experiment on your own with fasting or near-fasting if you inject insulin. If you have diabetes and want to try fasting or an FMD, work with your endocrinologist or reach out to scientists or hospitals establishing clinical trials.

CHAPTER 7

NEURODEGENERATIVE DISEASES

THE PROTEINS IN YOUR HEAD

When it comes to conditions associated with aging, neurodegenerative diseases, such as Alzheimer's disease, amyotrophic lateral sclerosis (ALS), dementia, Huntington's disease, and Parkinson's disease, rank among the most terrifying. The possibility of losing your independence or even your sense of self is a bleak one. Anyone who has accompanied a loved one through the stages of Alzheimer's disease, which accounts for somewhere between 60 and 80 percent of all neurodegenerative diseases, knows the keen torment of watching someone lose basic functions, including the capacity to recall memories or recognize their family, as well as the lingering worry that the same bomb might be ticking in your own brain.[67]

Researchers think the autophagy lysosomal pathway may be especially important for neurodegenerative diseases, for which aging is a

---

67 Longo, *The Longevity Diet.*

major risk factor, because aging brings a marked "down-regulation of autophagy in the brain."[68] The very nature of brain cells makes them a special case. Unlike most cells, neurons are postmitotic; they don't divide. This means that misfolded or aggregating proteins are a bigger deal since they aren't "diluted" over time as happens with cells that divide. Imagine dropping food coloring into a tub you are filling with water. So long as the water continues to fill the tub, the dye will disperse, and the overall effect will be muted, maybe even negligible. Now imagine dropping the same amount of food coloring into a cereal bowl filled with water. That dye will disperse very little and probably color the water dramatically. It's the same way with problematic proteins in your brain. Since your brain cells don't divide, nothing is watering them down. If these build up, they can become pathogenic.[69]

For this reason, quality control and intracellular housekeeping are invaluable for removing misfolded and damaged proteins from brain cells, as well as proteins that naturally tend to clump together, such as those found with Alzheimer's disease (tau proteins)[70] or Parkinson's disease (alpha-synuclein proteins).[71] Abnormal deposits of proteins have definitely been linked to these neurodegenerative conditions, as well as to Huntington's disease, ALS, and frontotemporal dementia, leading scientists to hypothesize that "autophagy dysfunction is a common mechanism in neurodegenerative disease."[72]

And researchers believe there may be genetic ties between many neurodegenerative diseases and the genes that regulate autophagy: "Mutations in many different genes associated with different steps in autophagy have been linked to Alzheimer's, Parkinson's, or

68 Finkbeiner, "The Autophagy Lysosomal Pathway and Neurodegeneration," 3.
69 Kroemer, "Autophagy: A Druggable Process That Is Deregulated in Aging and Human Disease," 1–4.
70 Ohsumi, "Historical Landmarks of Autophagy Research," 9–23.
71 Shetty, "Emerging Anti-aging Strategies—Scientific Basis and Efficacy," 1165–84.
72 Finkbeiner, "The Autophagy Lysosomal Pathway and Neurodegeneration," 3.

Huntington's disease, as well as ALS, frontotemporal dementia, and others."[73] Of course the issue isn't just discrete mutations in *ATG* genes; experts say that even "subtle defects" in autophagy can produce age-related neurodegeneration.[74]

NEURON FIRING

The complex structure and function of brain cells also play into their unique relationship with autophagy. These cells have central cell bodies with long, tail-like projections called axons and branchy arms called dendrites. Neurons don't touch each other inside your brain. The spaces between them are called synapses, and these empty areas are just as crucial as the other parts of the brain circuitry.

In order to communicate with each other, neurons "fire" electric impulses across those synapses, releasing chemical messages, called neurotransmitters, through the axon "tail." Neighboring brain cells catch the message using their dendrite "arms," and then launch their own. Every time this happens, the neurons playing catch form pathways through the synapses to each other, until passing messages to each other become reflexive—like a well-worn groove. This is why doing things over and over makes that practiced thing easier over time.

It's tempting to picture this taking place in miniature since these cells fit inside your skull, but scientists note that neurons have an "elaborated morphology" with dendrites and axons able to clock in at a meter in length or even longer![75] When it comes to autophagy, the autophagosomes—the cargo ships of the cell program—form at the end of the axon and travel up all the way to the cell body for degrading, under-

---

73 Finkbeiner, "The Autophagy Lysosomal Pathway and Neurodegeneration," 3.

74 Maiuri, "Therapeutic Modulation of Autophagy: Which Disease Comes First?" 680–89.

75 Finkbeiner, "The Autophagy Lysosomal Pathway and Neurodegeneration," 3.

going protein changes, such as a pH drop, during the journey.[76] That's a much more complicated situation than, say, simply scooping up a misfolded protein in the cytoplasm and taking it a miniscule distance for processing, like with most cells.

CURES ON THE HORIZON?

Not surprisingly, research for a cure for neurodegeneration has been ongoing for years, and the uptick in interest in autophagy has only fueled that fire. There is good evidence that some autophagy enhancers, such as rapamycin and lithium, can reduce protein aggregates and potentially lead to new treatment options for neurodegeneration.[77]

Of course, the most direct method of upregulating autophagy is calorie restriction through fasting or near-fasting, and experts have observed that calorie restriction protects against neurodegenerative disorders in mice.[78] However, it's not that simple when it comes to treating humans. For one thing, these diseases usually show up in old age, particularly between the ages of 60 and 95, and fasting and low-calorie diets aren't recommended for people in this age bracket.[79] More broadly, while there is some evidence that enhancing autophagy boosts clearance of disease-causing proteins, researchers worry that by the time a neurodegenerative disease manifests symptoms, it may be too late to benefit from an autophagy-enhancing drug or other intervention.[80, 81]

---

76 Finkbeiner, "The Autophagy Lysosomal Pathway and Neurodegeneration," 3.

77 Shetty, "Emerging Anti-aging Strategies—Scientific Basis and Efficacy," 1165–84.

78 Mattson, "Impact of Intermittent Fasting on Health and Disease Processes," 46–58.

79 Longo, *The Longevity Diet.*

80 Finkbeiner, "The Autophagy Lysosomal Pathway and Neurodegeneration," 3.

81 Maiuri, "Therapeutic Modulation of Autophagy: Which Disease Comes First?" 680–89.

There are more sweeping questions about how to figure out autophagy modulation in these diseases, such as what part of the pathway is affected by mutations in *ATG* genes. For example, mutations in a specific gene that enables the autophagosome to fuse with the lysosome causes frontotemporal dementia – but enhancing autophagy under these circumstances could result in a bunch of autophagosomes hanging out in the brain with no way for the body to clear them.[82]

Another concern is that the most likely mechanism for inducing autophagy—blocking the path of the protein mTOR kinase—might upset the other pathways the protein regulates (such as protein translation) and also suppress the immune system. Besides this, it's tough to develop mTOR inhibitors that can even cross into the brain, so researchers specifically working on brain-based diseases may need autophagy modulators separate from this pathway altogether.[83]

Which is to say the most obvious thing: neuroscience is complicated. This is why researchers hope to figure out all the underlying mechanisms that cause neurodegenerative conditions. It's also why they say they need better assays and markers to bridge the distance between animal studies and human clinical trials. After all, this is your brain they're talking about.

PREVENTATIVE STRATEGIES

In many cases, the best option may be delaying or preventing neurodegeneration. For Alzheimer's disease, delaying the age of onset by just five years would cut the overall number of people with the disease by almost half.[84]

---

82   Finkbeiner, "The Autophagy Lysosomal Pathway and Neurodegeneration," 3.

83   Finkbeiner, 3.

84   Longo, *The Longevity Diet*.

And researchers say those preventive strategies need to happen well before clinical signs show up. This has led some experts to suggest that people with a family history of neurodegeneration should undergo genetic testing to assess risk. For example, the Alzheimer's-linked *apolipoprotein E* gene comes in three variants, or alleles: E2, E3, and E4. Each person inherits two copies of this gene, and if one (or both) of those is the E4 allele, the risk of Alzheimer's increases significantly. The E3 allele is neutral when it comes to risk, and the rarest variant (E2) actually lowers the risk of developing the disease. At least one scientist thinks this information could help identify people who should use preventive strategies to try to buffer the effect of their genes. However, the National Institutes of Health doesn't yet agree; they don't recommend genetic testing except in very specific circumstances, such as before participating in a clinical trial.

The decision to test your genes (or not) is a very personal one, but the existing strategies to prevent or delay neurodegeneration are available to you right now. These include:

- Fasting or FMDs, preferably in concert with a Mediterranean diet, which is mostly plant-based with relatively high consumption of fats from olive oil and nuts, frequent consumption of seafood, and reduced consumption of other animal proteins. The Mediterranean diet has been shown to decrease the risk of neurodegeneration by 13 percent[85]

- Dietary changes like minimizing animal products, consuming about 3 daily tablespoons of coconut oil, which contains medium-chain fatty acids that protect against dementia, and hefty doses of coffee (yes!), which may be protective against Alzheimer's at 3 to 4 cups per day (yes, yes!)[86]

---

85 Longo, *The Longevity Diet.*
86 Longo, *The Longevity Diet.*

- Exercise, especially aerobic options like cycling, running, or swimming

- Mental stimulation, such as reading, puzzles and games, and taking classes

THE TAKEAWAY

Neurodegenerative diseases are particularly associated with autophagy because of the structure and function of brain cells and, because these cells don't divide, those problems are a bigger deal. Unfortunately, once diagnosed, treating these conditions is difficult. People with a neurodegenerative disease—especially if they are over the age of 65— must be careful with fasting or near-fasting and should only do so under medical supervision. Autophagy-enhancing interventions such as fasting, FMDs, supplements, and exercise may be potent ways to prevent or delay the onset of neurodegeneration.

CHAPTER 8

CANCER

THE C WORD

Few diseases strike fear quite like cancer, and for people who have close friends or family who faced the disease or who are cancer survivors themselves, cancer can take on a powerful role in a way that few other medical conditions ever will. People don't just have cancer or treat cancer; they battle it. And those battles are hard-fought. This fight may cost pieces of yourself or require you to willingly inject poison. People who don't have cancer but who fear it—especially those with a family history of inherited types of cancer—may even consider removal of body parts and organs that feel like ticking time bombs.

Considering all that cancer takes from its victims and survivors, it makes sense that interested parties pour money into cancer research, hoping for a cure. In 2019 alone, the National Institutes of Health budgeted a whopping 6.6 billion dollars for studying cancer.[87]

---

87 National Institutes of Health. "Estimates of Funding for Various Research, Condition, and Disease Categories," US Department of Health and Human Services, 19 April 2019. https://report.nih.gov/categorical_spending.aspx.

What even is this thing that takes so much? Your body contains 100 million million cells. Those cells are always growing and dividing, but if even one begins to grow in an out-of-control way—that's cancer. Benign tumors stay put and only cause problems if they press on important areas, like your brain. Malignant tumors spread, invading the surrounding tissues and even metastasizing, using your bloodstream like a highway to travel through your body and invade other organs.

A TROUBLING PARADOX

Since cancer cells are characterized by unrestrained growth, it seems logical that a cell program that eliminates malfunctioning cells would be just the ticket to override tumor formation. And that's true...sometimes. Autophagy can inhibit tumors by dealing with DNA damage and genome instability, but it can also encourage tumor growth in some cases. Because cancer is all about rapid cell growth, the energy demands of cancer cells are super steep. Hijacking the autophagy program, which recycles cell components into available energy, is a clever way for cancer cells to get the energy boost they need to proliferate. Some tumors can even exploit the program to survive cancer treatments like chemotherapy and radiation.[88] In some cases, blocking autophagy can sensitize cancer cells and make them more receptive to treatment.

Scientists call this seeming contradiction "paradoxical roles" and, as you might imagine, it makes figuring out the best way to leverage autophagy against cancer tricky. For any given tumor, the role of autophagy may be neutral, tumor-suppressing, or tumor-promoting.

---

88   Byun, "Therapeutic Implications of Autophagy Inducers in Immunological Disorders, Infection, and Cancer," 1959–81.

Determining whether to trigger or block autophagy during cancer treatment would require scientists and health-care providers to look at the context, such as tumor type, cancer stage, and even what body tissues are affected, and figure out what precise role autophagy plays in that particular tumor.[89]

One team of researchers speculates that this may be why about two-thirds of current clinical trials for cancer patients are looking at autophagy.[90] "Ultimately, pharmacologic manipulation of autophagy for cancer prevention and treatment will depend on the ability to successfully recognize the functional status of autophagy in tumors and on the availability of specific autophagy modulators," they say. It might even push oncology teams to personalize treatments plans. "It is important to determine whether, when, and how to block autophagy... to predict the use of autophagy in clinical settings for the treatment of cancer patients, to access the individual approach to cancer and its autophagy status."[91]

ALL THE WAY DOWN
THE RABBIT HOLE

In a paradox of the paradox, some researchers think the general stance on autophagy and cancer treatment—that is, blocking autophagy as the major hypothesis—may not tell the full, nuanced story. And following the thread of that tale leads to an underlying question of how cancer begins in the first place: "This debate—should we inhibit or

---

89 Byun, "Therapeutic Implications of Autophagy Inducers in Immunological Disorders, Infection, and Cancer," 1959–81.

90 Udristioiu, "Autophagy Dysfunctions Associated with Cancer Cells and Their Therapeutic Implications."

91 Udristioiu, "Autophagy Dysfunctions Associated with Cancer Cells and Their Therapeutic Implications."

enhance autophagy for cancer treatment?—is fueled by rather distinct visions of tumor pathogenesis."[92]

The traditional view that tumors arise as a result of genetic or epigenetic changes in cancer cells already underwent some tweaking after new information emerged about the immune system. It seems that tumors only show up when immunosurveillance fails, and anticancer treatments such as chemo or radiation only work long term if they also restore that immunosurveillance check.[93]

Some researchers have also shown that fasting or fast-mimicking diets, which trigger autophagy, undertaken before undergoing chemotherapy may protect against the side effects of the treatment and also enhance the effect of chemo.[94] This is, of course, the opposite of the statement you read five paragraphs ago, which gives you insight into just how tricky the autophagy/cancer dilemma is, even to scientists elbows deep in research.

One such expert, Valter Longo, describes autophagy-enhancing fasts before cancer treatments as a "magic shield," protecting healthy cells and immune cells from the damage of cancer treatment while leaving the tumor cells open to its assault. The idea jives with the theoretical observation that "short pulses of autophagy induction (as opposed to a protracted enhancement) would be sufficient to ignite durable anticancer immune responses, if appropriately combined with chemotherapy, radiotherapy, or immunotherapy."[95]

That somewhat radical idea—that starving cancer patients before treatment might improve clinical outcomes—has been the subject of animal studies and clinical trials for some time. The preliminary

92 Maiuri, "Therapeutic Modulation of Autophagy: Which Disease Comes First?" 680–89.

93 Maiuri, 680–89.

94 Longo, *The Longevity Diet.*

95 Maiuri, "Therapeutic Modulation of Autophagy: Which Disease Comes First?" 680–89.

results—notably for breast, colorectal, glioma, lung, melanoma, meso-thelioma, neuroblastoma, pancreatic, and prostate cancers—were so promising that the researchers secured NIH funding to develop a four-day pre-chemotherapy FMD specific for patients with cancer.[96]

OUNCE OF PREVENTION
> POUND OF CURE

Obviously, it would be better to avoid cancer altogether, and disease prevention is where autophagy shines. Autophagy acts as a barrier, pro-tecting against abnormal or damaged proteins and organelles in your cells.[97] It's only when the autophagy cell program breaks down that disease has an opportunity to take hold. And cancer is a tough adver-sary, always looking for that foothold. Some scientists describe cancer cells as "abnormally fit," like super villains who have developed the ability to break away from all the tumor-suppressing mechanisms in your cells as well as the surveillance activities of your immune system.[98]

When it comes to cancer prevention and FMDs, Longo recommends using an FMD for about a week every one to six months, depend-ing on how healthy you perceive yourself to be. Fastidious eaters and exercisers who maintain their bodies at peak fitness would fast or use the FMD only twice a year; people who struggle to follow eat-ing guidelines or who don't exercise would fast as often as one week per month. The effects appear to build over time with each round of FMD, so it's important to keep at it as part of a long-term lifestyle change. Longo also points out that people who know they are genet-ically predisposed to specific cancers, such as those who have *BRCA*

---

96 Longo, *The Longevity Diet*.

97 Byun, "Therapeutic Implications of Autophagy Inducers in Immunological Disorders, Infection, and Cancer," 1959–81.

98 Maiuri, "Therapeutic Modulation of Autophagy: Which Disease Comes First?" 680–89.

genes, which significantly increase the risk for developing breast cancer, should consider fasting protocols as something to try in addition to standard prophylactic procedures, such as mastectomy, and not as a replacement.

All people concerned about cancer, and especially those whose family or personal histories place them at higher risk for developing certain cancers, benefit from the role autophagy plays in keeping cells clear of potentially troublesome cell matter, including cell components that have the potential to develop into tumors. Since natural interventions that trigger autophagy also support a robust immune system—and the immune system monitors for cancers—those two autophagy-dependent functions (clearing the cells and supporting immune response) seem to position autophagy as a way to bolster the body against any future battle with cancer.

THE TAKEAWAY

Once cancer shows up, autophagy can go either way when it comes to suppressing tumor growth or giving tumors a boost. The decision to modulate autophagy in conjunction with typical treatment, such as chemotherapy or radiation, likely depends on complex factors, including the type of tumor, stage of cancer, and the tissues involved. It also depends on which scientists you talk to since the question is still being debated.

If you have cancer and want to explore using autophagy to enhance treatment, talk with your health-care provider or reach out to researchers, such as the Valter Longo Foundation, or research hospitals involved in autophagy-related clinical trials. It's not a good idea to embark on a pre-chemo fasting plan without the knowledge and guidance of a health-care provider.

If you are concerned about your family history of cancer or just hope to avoid the disease, autophagy-enhancing lifestyle choices, such as fasting, exercise, and consuming foods with pro-autophagic benefits (check out all these options in Part III) may help your body clear the abnormal cell components that could one day become cancer. They may also boost your immune system, which plays a role in fighting cancer cells that do show up.

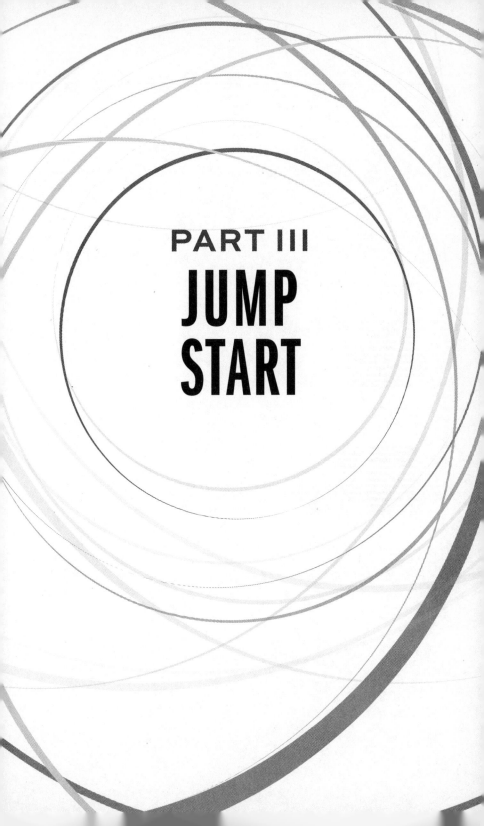

PART III
JUMP START

CHAPTER 9

FASTING

STARVE FOR YOUR HEALTH

As you know, your autophagy program is a stress response conserved by evolution to help you survive when resources dry up. Should you find yourself waiting out a nuclear winter in a bunker, living on canned pears and rat steaks, autophagy will helpfully kick in and recycle nonessential proteins and organelles. This allows your cells to save energy on synthesis and siphons usable energy from some of the rejected cellular debris. On the flip side, the fact that most people never experience starvation conditions means that they have the opposite problem: too many calories and the potential for a sluggish baseline program.

For science and health enthusiasts interested in tapping into the benefits of the autophagy program, the solution is straightforward: Trick your body into exercising its stress response. According to the experts, the most efficient methods to do that—and therefore postpone aging and avoid disease—are calorie restriction, calorie restriction mimetics, and exercise.[99] Those same experts point out that traditional or folk medicines have long prescribed these very tools to promote longevity

99 Maiuri, "Therapeutic Modulation of Autophagy: Which Disease Comes First?" 680–89.

and improved health span, recognizing the benefits of the autophagy program well before science uncovered the cellular mechanisms. And while there is no doubt a market for pharmacological agents like pills and prescriptions that modulate autophagy, the jury is still out on whether those preparations will ever be as effective as the natural options.

FASTING FOR THE GODS

Most religions and spiritual traditions include some type of fasting protocol in their practices, and many human-based studies of fasting look at populations who fast regularly for this reason. For example, practitioners of Islam who fast during Ramadan are a pretty common source of data for researchers interested in the effects of fasting.

Here's a quick and dirty list of religions that incorporate fasting for spiritual benefit:

- Ancient Hellenistic mystery religions
- Baha'i
- Buddhism
- Christianity, including Roman Catholicism and the Latter Day Saints
- Hinduism
- Indigenous religions
- Islam
- Jainism
- Judaism
- Paganism and witchcraft
- Taoism

One of the very few exceptions to this is Zoroastrianism, which discourages or even prohibits fasting.

WHAT IS CALORIE RESTRICTION?

According to the National Institutes of Health, calorie restriction (CR) means "reducing average daily caloric intake below what is typical or habitual without malnutrition or deprivation of essential nutrients."[100] CR is easy to establish in the laboratory using research animals who generally receive a single daily feeding. For these animals, who form the basis of much of the research on the benefits of fasting, this means reducing the daily food allotment by 10 to 40 percent.

Calorie restriction and fasting often overlap, but they aren't the same thing. CR focuses on reducing the calories you eat during the day while fasting focuses on limiting the frequency of eating. This means that a person (or lab rat) who fasts might also engage in CR simply because less feeding time likely means fewer calories, but not necessarily.

When it comes to autophagy, these periodic breaks in calorie consumption jump start the cell program, which has been programmed by evolution to recognize starvation as an on switch. Of all the autophagy-enhancing options, calorie restriction and/or fasting are the most effective. Researchers say CR activates multiple autophagy-regulating pathways, and fasting has been linked to improvements in the human health span, including addressing conditions like cardiovascular and metabolic diseases and cancer. [101, 102]

And don't worry, you won't die. At any given time, you have around 10,000 calories stored in your body, ready to provide the energy to keep you going, even if you don't put anything in your mouth.

---

100   National Institute on Aging. "Calorie Restriction and Fasting Diets: What Do We Know?" National Institutes of Health. (2018) www.nia.nih.gov/health/calorie-restriction-and-fasting-diets-what-do-we-know.

101   Madeo, "Essential Role for Autophagy in Life Span Extension," 85–93.

102   Madeo, 85–93.

FASTING FOR THE SOCIAL GOOD

Any discussion of fasting would be incomplete without addressing one of its oldest uses: as a means of nonviolent protest. Here are some of the most famous or notable hunger strikes.

First reference to fasting: According to a subplot of the epic Sanskrit poem *Ramayana* (circa 300 BCE), a king had four sons. The mother of the second son, Bharata, schemed to have the eldest, Rama, exiled so that her own son could ascend to the throne. When the king died, Bharata, who was tight with his exiled brother, placed his brother's slippers on the throne as a symbol that he was only a stand-in leader until his elder brother returned. He then abdicated royal luxuries, spending the next 14 years in the nearby forest, eating only roots and praying.

Interesting legal reference: Pre-Christian Irish law recognized that people with high social ranks could wrong those beneath them. To redress a wrong, the victim could sit outside the wrongdoer's home and fast to curse the perp. The householder had two options: admit the wrong and make amends, which would end the fast and expunge the bad luck, or counter-fast to avoid the curse without admitting wrong. Even more interesting, St. Patrick supposedly invoked this ancient law against the Christian God, who had refused some of St. Patrick's demands, notably his not-at-all-egotistical demand that he should weigh the Irish souls at final judgment in God's place. The saint climbed the local holy mountain and fasted there for 40 days and nights—reportedly in a foul mood and singing malicious songs the whole time—until God conceded.

Famous fasts: Mohandas Gandhi undertook multiple fasts for social change, especially addressing home rule and the Indian caste system. His most famous (and longest) fast began January 12, 1948. Across the pond, United Farm Workers leader Cesar Chavez fasted to bring attention to the plight of farm workers, who suffered terrible working conditions and low pay. His most famous fast in 1968 lasted for 25 days, drawing the attention of leaders including Martin Luther King Jr. and Robert Kennedy. Other famous hunger strikes include many instances of prisoners refusing food to bring attention to injustices or conditions, notably in Northern Ireland, Palestine, and the US. Suffragettes in both the UK and US have refused to eat until they secured the right to vote.

Longest fast: This distinction goes to Chanu Sharmila, who refused food and water for 16 years hoping to end an Indian law that gave deadly authority to local armed forces. Sharmila was routinely arrested and force-fed during that time, until she ended her hunger strike and entered politics in 2016.

SO MANY FASTS, SO LITTLE TIME

When most people think about fasting, they probably picture historical photos of hunger strikers or religious ascetics and long periods of putting exactly nothing in your mouth. And that's certainly one option. Experts call these periodic fasts or prolonged fasting (PF), and they look like cycles of normal eating interspersed with periods of simply not eating. Usually the periodic fast lasts 24 to 48 hours, but some practitioners choose to fast for two or more days at a time with a solid week of normal-eating recovery between PF cycles. When it comes to autophagy, these longer cycles of fasting (two or more days in a row) are ideal for triggering the cell program and racking up the health benefits.[103] This ideal window may be reduced to 24 hours in some studies and circumstances.[104]

That's all fine and good, and if the stringent schedule of periodic fasting works for you, rock on. It's a tough sell for people accustomed to shoveling food into their mouths every few hours, though, and the added pressures of lives with kids and careers make it even harder to stick with it. Have you ever tried to just not eat for two days while making a million meals and snacks for toddlers? It's tough.

The friendlier alternative is intermittent fasting (IF), which exploits the benefits of fasting while minimizing the downsides of prolonged fasting. To do this, IF sets windows for eating and windows for fasting. Research suggests that this strategy is just as effective as traditional fasting: "Restricting the timing of food intake to a few hours without an overt attempt to reduce caloric intake may trigger the fasting physiology after a few hours of feeding cessation on a daily basis."[105] If intermittent fasting sounds right for you, you have lots of options. The most common are the 16/8 method and the 5:2 plan.

THE 16/8 METHOD

To do this, restrict your daily eating to an 8-hour window of your choosing. This technique is also called time-restricted eating (TRE) when used by researchers as a form of calorie restriction in animal studies. The science behind the method hinges on the idea of circadian

---

103   Sebastian Brandhorst et al. "A Periodic Diet That Mimics Fasting Promotes Multi-system Regeneration, Enhanced Cognitive Performance, and Health Span," *Cell Metabolism* 22 (2015): 88–99. https://doi.org/10.1016/j.cmet.2015.05.012.

104   Mehrdad Alirezael et al. "Short-term Fasting Induces Profound Neuronal Autophagy," *Autophagy* 6, no. 6 (2010): 702–10. https://doi.org/10.4161/auto.6.6.12376.

105   Valter Longo and Satchidananda Panda. "Fasting, Circadian Rhythms, and Time Restricted Feeding in Healthy Life Span," *Cell Metabolism* 23, no. 6 (2016): 1048–59. https://doi.org/10.1016/j.cmet.2016.06.001.

plasticity. Before electricity and artificial light became a thing, humans probably only ate during natural daylight and fasted during the dark hours simply because scavenging or feeding in the pitch black was dangerous.[106]

According to circadian rhythm theories, the introduction of artificial light disrupted the internal clock that governs sleep/wake cycles and activities, resulting in overfed, sleep-deprived humans. You probably already fast while you're sleeping your solid 8 to 9 hours per night (ha ha), so the 16/8 method just stretches that fasting window to 16 hours and shortens the eating window to 8 hours. Functionally, this can look like skipping breakfast and setting your feeding window for noon to 8 pm. Breakfast lovers, don't despair; the positioning of the window doesn't matter, so you can choose to eat from 9 a.m. to 5 p.m. (or whenever you want).

While the internet is brimming with additional rules and ideas, the only real regulation here is to restrict eating to 8 hours. That's it.

THE 5:2 PLAN

The 5:2 plan is like the weekly version of time-restricted eating. To do this, reduce your intake to 500 to 600 calories on each of two non-consecutive days in the week, and eat normally on the other five. The benefit here is that most of the week is just normal eating, so any downsides that come with CR (like feeling grumpier than usual or needing to plan social events around your fast) happen only on the days you selected. The science here is pretty sound, at least for insects.

---

106   Longo, "Fasting, Circadian Rhythms, and Time Restricted Feeding in Healthy Life Span," 1048–59.

One month of this diet at the beginning of adulthood extended the life span of fruit flies and reduced age-related pathologies.[107]

LESS COMMON OPTIONS

And, of course, there are other ways to fast intermittently, such as:

Eat-Stop-Eat: Fast 24 hours once or twice per week. Practitioners of this type of fasting nest it under IF, although it is very similar to the lower end of periodic fasting.

Alternate-Day Fasting: Reduce intake to 0 to 25 percent of your usual calories every other day.

Warrior Diet: Fast 20 hours, then binge 4 hours. This is really IF cranked up to its max. The designer of the method, Ori Hofmekler, believes it models the likely eating patterns of Paleolithic people.

SOME IMPORTANT CAVEATS

Fasting isn't for everybody. It's not a good idea for people who are pregnant or nursing, children and adolescents, extreme athletes, people who are underweight or have preexisting health conditions (talk to your health-care provider), people with eating disorders or a history of disordered eating, or people over 65. There seem to be some differences linked to sex assignment in the effects of fasting, so people hoping to become pregnant—or who have reproductive or endocrine concerns—should consult with a health-care provider or nutrition expert.

---

107 Shetty, "Emerging Anti-aging Strategies—Scientific Basis and Efficacy," 1165–84.

SO, WHAT'S THE BEST FAST?

There really is no "best" option since your ideal fast is based on highly personal factors, such as your lifestyle and reasons for fasting. It makes sense to pick one fasting technique and stick with it long enough to experience the benefits of fasting, probably a solid month or longer. Look for specific fasting recommendations hitting the health consumer sphere in the next few years as scientists and health-care providers begin leveraging the research into actionable diets, personalized for specific diseases and conditions.

CHAPTER 10

ALTERNATIVE FASTING DIETS

YOU ARE WHAT YOU EAT

Prolonged and intermittent fasting aren't the only options. Other eating styles—some trendy, some not so much—may also tap into the benefits of the autophagy lysosomal pathway without the downsides that come with triggering your starvation response, such as inconvenience and minor physical discomforts associated with hunger. While PF and IF focus on *when* you eat, these alternative techniques pay attention to *what* you eat.

LOW-PROTEIN DIETS

There are four types of large molecules (macromolecules) that make life possible: carbohydrates, lipids, nucleic acids, and proteins. One way to trick your body into triggering the starvation response without actually starving yourself is to substantially lower just one macromolecule:

protein. A low-protein diet, which means deriving less than 10 percent of your daily calories from protein, may be a good way to do this. According to one study, people under 65 may be able to minimize the risk of age-related diseases and mortality just by laying off the burgers (and other high-protein foods).[108] This is because "low protein consumption in humans and mice is associated with reduced risk for age-related diseases and mortality, probably through reduced signaling of IGF-1, which is an important negative regulator of autophagy."[109]

One simple way to meet this low-protein goal is to adopt a vegetarian or vegan diet, since eliminating meat and/or dairy necessarily reduces animal protein. One study found that vegans consumed about 82 grams of protein daily compared with 112 grams for omnivores (and 93 grams for vegetarians). They reported significant overall decreases in total calories, too. Vegans and vegetarians self-reported around 2,400 and 2,700 calories, respectively, while meat eaters clocked in at almost 3,000 calories.[110] All of these were higher than the general recommended guideline of 7 grams of protein per 20 pounds of body weight, so you would still need to track and count your protein intake to make sure you stay under the 10 percent threshold.[111]

If saying goodbye to chicken nuggets and milkshakes is just too much, consider a protein fast. This alternative fasting diet focuses on carefully regulating protein consumption for 24 hours without overall calorie restriction. Most people who use protein fasting eat no (or very low) protein and low carb for the 24-hour fast, focusing on consuming

---

108 Morgan E. Levine et al. "Low Protein Intake Is Associated with a Major Reduction in Igf-1, Cancer, and Overall Mortality in the 65 and Younger but Not Older Population," *Cell Metabolism* 19, no. 3 (2014): 407–17. https://doi.org/10.1016/j.cmet.2014.02.006.

109 Madeo, "Essential Role for Autophagy in Life Span Extension," 85–93.

110 Peter Clarys et al. "Comparison of Nutritional Quality of the Vegan, Vegetarian, Semi-Vegetarian, Pesco-Vegetarian, and Omnivorous Diet," *Nutrients* 6, no. 3 (2014): 1318–32. https:/doi: 10.3390/nu6031318.

111 Harvard School of Public Health. "The Nutrition Source: Protein." https://www.hsph .harvard.edu/nutritionsource/what-should-you-eat/protein.

mostly fats. The most hardcore adherents protein cycle, which means protein fasting one day followed by a high-protein recovery day.

THE KETOGENIC DIET

Unless you've been living under a rock for the past few years, you've probably heard the term keto. This diet actually started as a clinical treatment for epilepsy beginning in the 1920s. The traditional clinical macro breakdown for keto diets is 3:1 (sometimes 4:1) grams of fat to grams of protein and carbohydrates.[112] This usually shakes out to 75 percent of daily calories from fat, 20 percent of daily calories from protein, and 5 percent of daily calories from carbs. With the evolving of the keto diet from clinical applications (like epilepsy) to self-health populations, those percentages have evolved, too. Some keto adherents derive anywhere from 5 to 25 percent of daily calories from protein. And there's always the option to cycle keto, or take intentional breaks from the keto diet once or twice a week (or at other regular intervals).

FAST-MIMICKING DIETS

One scientist author, Valter Longo, crafted what he calls a longevity diet.[113] This fasting-mimicking diet (FMD) limits the amount of time spent fasting (or near fasting) to just a few times per year while promising similar results in terms of health span.

---

112   Adam L. Hartman and Eileen P. G. Vining. "Clinical Aspects of the Ketogenic Diet," *Epilepsia* 48, no. 1 (2007): 31–42. https://doi.org/10.1111/j.1528-1167.2007.00914.x.

113   Longo, *The Longevity Diet*.

Longo's fast-mimicking diet looks like this:

Day 1: 1,100 calories, including 500 calories from complex carbohydrate vegetables (like broccoli, pumpkin, mushrooms, and tomatoes), 500 calories from fats (olive oil and nuts), 25 grams of plant-based protein (nuts), a multivitamin, mineral and omega-3/omega-6 supplements, up to 4 cups of sugarless tea, unlimited water

Days 2 through 5: 800 calories, half from complex carb veggies and half from healthy fats, a multivitamin and supplements, up to 4 cups of sugarless tea, unlimited water

Day 6 (transition to normal eating): focus on complex carbohydrates, such as vegetables, pasta, rice, bread, and fruit, and minimize fish and saturated fats, such as meat, milk, cheese, desserts

To make this FMD easier and for the purposes of using it in the lab, Longo developed an FMD-in-a-box option called ProLon, which enables consumers to try out FMD without piecing it together themselves. Longo donates the proceeds from this product to research.

The intriguing thing about Longo's longevity diet (other than his impressive scientific pedigree) is that he has used his FMD in both animal studies and human clinical trials. In fact, he developed his diet after trying out a fasting regimen with cancer patients, which he says had good clinical results but just wasn't feasible since the patients were basically miserable. This inspired Longo to figure out a way to mimic fasting without the downsides.

When Longo used a three-day FMD on middle-aged mice, he reported good results. They lived longer, preserved bone mineral density, reduced incidence of skin inflammatory disorders, increased levels of stem cells, and performed better on cognitive tests as they aged. When it comes to cancer, the FMD-fed mice wound up with half the expected number of tumors and delayed onset of cancer for the equivalent of about 10 human years. The tumors that did show up in FMD-fed mice were not widespread in the affected animals, which Longo says suggests they were benign.

Longo found these results remarkable and turned to human subjects. In the randomized study of 100 patients, participants used an FMD for five days per month for three months total. He reported decreases in fasting glucose, blood pressure, cholesterol, triglycerides, and measures associated with cancer (IGF-1) and cardiovascular disease (c-reactive protein). Even more exciting for Longo, the subjects continued to see those changes three months after returning to their normal diets, causing him to assert that using his five-day FMD program every three months might reduce the risk of many of the diseases associated with aging.

Longo isn't the only researcher using fast-mimicking diets, either. In a separate clinical trial, participants cycled a proprietary plant-based diet, resulting in decreased markers for aging, cancer, cardiovascular disease, and diabetes.[114] This diet was tightly controlled by the study and included three cycles like this:

Day 1: 1,090 calories: 10 percent protein, 56 percent fat, 34 percent carbs

Days 2 to 5: 725 calories: 9 percent protein, 44 percent fat, 47 percent carbs

Another clinical trial looked at the effects of an FMD on multiple sclerosis (MS). The authors found that a seven-day FMD followed by six

---

114 Brandhorst, "A Periodic Diet That Mimics Fasting Promotes Multisystem Regeneration, Enhanced Cognitive Performance, and Health Span," 88–99.

months of a Mediterranean diet had positive outcomes for patients with MS.[115]

Overall, "CR or various other dietary restrictions and particularly relatively long-term fasting, or FMD cycles followed by refeeding appear to decrease the biological rate of aging and promote anti-inflammatory effects—and may contribute to alleviate and possibly reverse a variety of autoimmune disorders as well as immune-senescence by killing old and damaged cells and replacing them with young and functional ones."[116] The diseases specifically noted here include asthma, lupus, multiple sclerosis, and rheumatoid arthritis.

115   In Young Choi et al. "A Diet Mimicking Fasting Promotes Regeneration and Reduces Autoimmunity and Multiple Sclerosis Symptoms," *Cell Reports* 15, no. 10 (2016): 2136-46. https://doi.org/10.1016/j.celrep.2016.05.009.

116   In Young Choi et al. "Nutrition and Fasting Mimicking Diets in the Prevention and Treatment of Autoimmune Diseases and Immunosenescence," *Molecular and Cellular Endocrinology* 455 (2017): 4–12. https://doi.org/10.1016/j.mce.2017.01.042.

CHAPTER 11

EXERCISE

BURN SOME ENERGY

There are many reasons that fasting and fasting alternatives might not work for everybody or every body. That's okay! You don't have to throw in the towel and succumb to stockpiling old proteins in your cells like some sort of a molecular hoarder. Starvation isn't the only way to trigger your stress response.

Scientists believe exercise also kicks up the autophagy program since muscle contraction is another form of stress. Scientists first observed the purported link between autophagy and exercise in the 1980s when they noticed that the size and number of autophagic vacuoles in the liver and skeletal muscle tissues of exercised lab animals increased in comparison with sedentary control animals. Some experts think exercise may even be "a more potent physiological method to induce autophagy in a short period of time," at least in lab mice. This makes sense because studies suggest that fasting is most effective in lab mice around the 48-hour time point, which is a very long time for most humans to fast or use calorie restriction in real life. Those same researchers can trigger the autophagy lysosomal pathway in lab mice in as little as 30 minutes of treadmill running.[117]

Another group of experts who compared exercise outcomes with other autophagy inducers, such as pharmaceuticals and nutritional changes, believe regular exercise may be the most effective option for upping the autophagy program. They say that a long-term (think: life-long) aerobic exercise regimen dampened some age-related features: the decline in autophagy proteins seen with normal aging, age-related increases in oxidative damage, and incidence of programmed cell death (called apoptosis).[118]

RUN (OR SWIM OR BIKE) AWAY FROM OLD AGE

Exercise has been shown to diminish the nine hallmarks of aging.[119] These are basically what being old means, as viewed through a scientific lens, and these features show up when researchers trigger premature aging.

They include:[120]

Genomic instability: the buildup of genetic damage, which happens over the course of your life, thanks to DNA-damaging exposures,

---

117   Altea Rocchi and Congcong He. "Activating Autophagy By Aerobic Exercise in Mice," *Journal of Visualized Experiments* 120 (2017): e55099. https://doi.org/10.3791/55099.

118   Anna Vainshtein and David A. Hood. "The Regulation of Autophagy During Exercise in Skeletal Muscle," *Journal of Applied Physiology* 120, no. 6 (2016): 664–73. https://doi.org/10.1152/japplphysiol.00550.2015.

119   Nuria Garatachea et al. "Exercise Attenuates the Major Hallmarks of Aging," *Rejuvenation Research* 18, no. 1 (2015): 57–89. https://doi.org/10.1089/rej.2014.1623.

120   Carlos Lopez-Otin et al. "The Hallmarks of Aging," *Cell* 153 (2013): 1194-1217. https://doi.org/10.1016/j.cell.2013.05.039.

replication errors, and spontaneous chemical reactions that happen inside your cells

Telomere attrition: the end sections of your chromosomes (tasked with preventing deterioration or fusing with neighbor chromosomes) simply wearing out

Epigenetic alterations: theoretically reversible changes to genes (for instance, adding a methyl group) that can act like on/off switches for those genes and which may accumulate with age

Loss of proteostasis: out-of-balance quality control for protein folding and degradation; this includes your autophagy lysosomal pathway

Deregulated nutrient-sensing: the decrease in the ability of your cells to recognize and respond to molecules like glucose, which involves autophagy-linked pathways

Mitochondrial dysfunction: reduces the ability of these organelles to produce the energy your cells need and regulate cell metabolism, which relies on a type of autophagy (mitophagy)

Cellular senescence: cells becoming unable to divide

Stem cell exhaustion: decline in stem cells available and able to differentiate into the cells your body uses to repair tissues

Altered intercellular communication: changes in the cell's ability to communicate, resulting in inflammation and/or reduced immunosurveillance

Researchers think some of these features may explain the neuroprotective effects of exercise, which (especially in the form of aerobic endurance training) significantly benefits people with Alzheimer's disease. Of course, it also positively addresses sarcopenia, the loss of muscle and strength that often accompanies old age. This condition affects 5 to 13 percent of people in their 60s and up to half of people over age 80.[121]

BUT HOW MUCH EXERCISE?

From ancient Greece right up to the present moment, humans have been generally prone to admire their most athletic peers. You probably watch them work, cheer them on, and even consider it a patriotic undertaking (oh, hi Olympics) in some cases. And don't forget the urge to buy the products they endorse and wear replicas of their uniforms. It turns out these elite athletes aren't just well-paid and beloved; they also enjoy considerably longer lives than the regular population.[122]

That's all fine and good, but Olympians and other elite athletes work out for their jobs, and average people don't have 25 hours a week (or more) to dedicate to exercise. So, what's enough?

One of the first studies that linked autophagy to exercise used mice engineered so that their autophagosomes glowed bright green to help visualize the effects of exercise on autophagy. Those researchers found that the number of autophagosomes in both skeletal and cardiac muscle increased—which means autophagy was turned and on and taking up cell matter for recycling—after just 30 minutes of treadmill running. These numbers plateaued after the mice had been running for 80 minutes.[123] When looking at the green glowing tissues of the mice, the researchers also noted an upregulation in autophagy in the

---

121   Garatachea, "Exercise Attentuates the Major Hallmarks of Aging," 57–89.

122   Garatachea, 57–89.

123   C. He et al. "Exercise-Induced BCL2-Regulated Autophagy Is Required for Muscle Glucose Homeostasis," *Nature* 481, no. 7382 (2012): 511–15. https://doi.org/10.1038/nature10758.

liver and pancreas (which both influence glucose and energy) as well as adipose tissue.

When it comes to humans, researchers have quantified precisely how much exercise correlates with longevity—without regard for the cellular mechanisms underlying the results—by comparing self-reported physical activity with 14 years' worth of death records.[124] They found that the sweet spot (or Goldilocks zone, as in juuuust right) is somewhere between 150 and 450 minutes of exercise per week. Moderate exercisers at the lower end of that scale who crank out about an hour of exertion three times a week reportedly reduced their risk of premature death by 31 percent. Folks who laced up their sneakers a whopping 450 minutes per week, which is about an hour a day, every day, if you're keeping count, reduced their risk of early death by an impressive 39 percent.

Of course, it's impossible to link this research data conclusively to the autophagy lysosomal pathway. However, another study reported that a single bout of exercise (about 60 minutes of moderate cycling) increased the number of autophagosomes in study participants. Doing this three times per week for an eight-week training period also increased autophagic markers.[125] So, while this is most definitely not a call to jump to conclusions, it's also not a huge leap.

Remember those mice with the autophagosomes that glow green? One of the researchers was so struck by the study results that he bought a treadmill, which is compelling all by itself. Here's some more good news: The human longevity study noted that people who exercise regularly but don't quite meet that 150 minutes per week benchmark still

124   Hannah Arem et al. "Leisure Time Physical Activity and Mortality: A Detailed Pooled Analysis of the Dose-Response Relationship," *JAMA Internal Medicine* 175, no. 6 (2015): 959–67. https://doi.org/10.1001/jamainternmed.2015.0533.

125   Nina Brandt et al. "Exercise and Exercise-Training Induced Increase in Autophagy Markers in Human Skeletal Muscle," *Physiological Reports* 6, no. 7 (2018): e13651. https://doi.org/10.14814/phy2.13651.

reduce their risk of premature death by 20 percent when compared with people who don't exercise at all.

UPPING YOUR GAME

Experts who study the link between exercise and human longevity also point out that the life span–improving benefits aren't just about clocking minutes. If you can push yourself from the moderate exercise zone into the vigorous exercise zone for around 30 percent of your total workout, you can grab an extra 9 to 13 percent reduction in mortality.[126] If you're exercising at the lower end of the guideline, that translates to three 50-minute workouts with 15 minutes of high intensity exercise per session.

You can even make this your whole exercise strategy. High-intensity interval training (HIIT) alternates spurts of intense exercise with less intense recovery periods until you reach the point of exhaustion. The resultant excess post-exercise oxygen consumption (EPOC)—or afterburn effect—means that the benefits of the workout linger much longer than with plain old moderate exercise. This is likely true for the autophagy-related benefits of exercise, too.

One group of researchers found that rats that exercised using HIIT strategies saw improved physical performance and an amped up baseline autophagy program compared with rats on a regular moderate intensity exercise regimen.[127] A year later, those same researchers measured endurance, the number of autophagosomes, and protein expression in a group of rats performing HIIT workouts. While both

---

126   Arem, "Leisure Time Physical Activity and Mortality: A Detailed Pooled Analysis of the Dose-Response Relationship," 959–67.

127   Fang-Hui Li et al. "Beneficial Autophagic Activities, Mitochondrial Function, and Metabolic Phenotype Adaptations Promoted by High-Intensity Interval Training in a Rat Model." *Frontiers in Physiology* 9 (2018): 571. https://doi.org/10.3389/fphys.2018.00571.

moderate exercisers and HIIT rats saw improvements compared with the control rats who did not exercise, the rats on the HIIT program activated pathways important for autophagy (such as the mTOR pathway), altered the expression of proteins important for breaking down and rebuilding proteins, and enhanced autophagy in specific muscles.[128] A similar study looking only at aged female rats reported similar benefits and suggested that HIIT may be particularly beneficial for those initiating an exercise program late in life, since the protocol improved age-related issues with the autophagy program via the AMPK/FOXO pathway.[129]

Even better news: It seems likely that combining autophagic triggers, such as using regular exercise with periodic fasting or near-fasting protocols plus including foods rich in CR mimetics in your diet, could have an additive result. One study already found that consuming the antioxidant spermidine and performing moderate exercise, such as swimming 60 minutes per day, five days per week, may be even more effective than doing either of those things alone. The lab mice who ate spermidine and swam reversed the age-related atrophy of skeletal muscle—via the mechanism of autophagy—within just 42 days.[130]

128   Xinwen Cui et al. "HIIT Changes the Expression of MuRF1 and MAFBx Proteins and Proteins Involved in the mTOR Pathway and Autophagy in Rat Skeletal Muscle." *Experimental Physiology* (2019). https://doi.org/10.1113/EP087601.

129   Fang-Hui Li et al. "Proteomics-Based Identification of Different Training Adaptations of Aged Skeletal Muscle Following Long-Term High-Intensity Interval and Moderate-Intensity Continuous Training in Aged Rats." *Aging* 11, no. 12 (2019): 4159–82. https://doi.org/10.18632/aging.102044

130   Jingjing Fan et al. "Spermidine Coupled with Exercise Rescues Skeletal Muscle Atrophy," *Oncotarget* 8, no. 11 (2017): 17475–90. https://doi.org/10.18632/oncotarget.15728.

CHAPTER 12

SUPPLEMENTS AND MIMETICS

TOO LONG; DIDN'T FAST

So what if fasting, fasting alternatives, and exercise all seem too oner-ous? You're in luck! Some compounds, including many that naturally occur in foods you probably already eat, trick your body into the auto-phagic benefits of fasting and exercise—without missing a meal or swimming a single lap. These are called CR mimetics or sometimes pro-autophagic components. A diet rich in these compounds just might amp up autophagy.

The pharmaceutical and natural health industries are well aware that a magic pill that imparts the benefits of autophagy would be a big deal for lots of people. It's no surprise that multiple industries are interested in monetizing pro-autophagic compounds. Researchers say that fig-uring out consumer-friendly packaged compounds that activate the autophagy lysosomal pathway the same way that calorie restriction does would be a major feat for public health. Public and private (both for- and not-for-profit) research organizations have already begun looking at several CR mimetics for this reason.

DRUGS, DRUGS, DRUGS

The pharmaceutical industry wants to meet the demands of a growing population of aging Americans who desire improved health spans along with their longer lives. One promising research area is repurposing well-known medications for new clinical applications. The most obvious benefit of this strategy is that these medications have established drug profiles, have already undergone clinical trials, and have already secured FDA approval. Expanding the label for other applications, such as aging or disease treatment, requires additional clinical trials but enables the drug to skip the phases associated with safety.

Some researchers are looking at the prescription drug metformin for possible rebranding as an anti-aging drug. This common medication for type 2 diabetes extends the life span of nematodes and rodents in the lab. It also stretches the health span of mice by reducing oxidative stress and inflammation. Its ability to attenuate tumor growth and possibly even protect against cancer is the subject of over 100 ongoing clinical studies.[131] Possible mechanisms include insulin-related activity, decreasing IGF-1 signaling (which is known to increase longevity in mammals), activation of AMP kinase (which coordinates autophagy), and inhibition of the mTOR pathway (preventing autophagy in lymphoma cells).

The immunosuppressant sirolimus (commonly called rapamycin) is currently used to prevent immune rejection after organ transplantation. The drug also increases the life span of lab mice and is in clinical trials

---

131 "Metformin in Longevity Study," National Institutes of Health US National Library of Medicine, Clinical Trials. https://clinicaltrials.gov/ct2/show/study/NCT02432287.

as an anti-aging medication. The likely mechanism is inhibition of the mTOR pathway. According to one researcher, self-administering sirolimus for anti-aging purposes is already happening in places with more relaxed pharmaceutical regulations.

Of course, as mentioned in an earlier chapter, the real money is in drug discovery; that is, looking for brand-new drugs that enhance or block autophagy. Experts say that any real drive to bring established drugs into the equation will require the investment of a public sponsor.

ANTIOXIDANTS AND OTHER NATURALLY OCCURRING COMPOUNDS

To make sense of the claims made by proponents of antioxidants, you'll need to travel back in your mind to chemistry class. In an atom, the protons and neutrons hang out in the center while the electrons orbit in a cloud. Atoms with a lot of electrons will have some at the outer edges, or shell, of that electron cloud. These are valence electrons, and nature likes to keep them paired up. Atoms with unpaired electrons in the outer shell are called free radicals, and these are unstable. They are desperate to fill their empty slots and do this by stealing electrons from stable atoms; chemists call this highly reactive.

One theory of aging is that free radicals, in their desperation to fill their shells, ultimately damage important biomolecules, and this damage accumulates as aging. This oxidative damage might be protected by— you guessed it—antioxidants. These compounds help protect plants from damaging conditions—stressors such as sun damage, extreme temperatures, drought, water that is too saline, or fungal diseases— since, unlike animals, plants are rooted in their spots and can't just walk away from environmental stress. And when you eat those plants, the antioxidants benefit your cells in the same way.

Here are some antioxidant compounds that trigger autophagy:

You might not know resveratrol by name, but you've probably heard about its benefits. It's the natural antioxidant found in grape skins and berries, which is responsible for the benefits of drinking red wine (thank you!) and is available as a dietary supplement. Some animal models link **resveratrol** with beneficial effects on Alzheimer's disease, blood sugar, cardiovascular conditions, and cancer.

Another well-known antioxidant is **curcumin**, which is found in the ginger-family spice turmeric and also as a dietary supplement. Curcumin has been shown to be anti-inflammatory and potentially anti-carcinogenic. In the lab, it extends the life span of round worms and fruit flies via antioxidative activity, including the autophagy-linked FOXO3 pathway, also called the human longevity genes.[132]

It's an unfortunate name, but the antioxidant **spermidine** (first found in semen, yikes) naturally occurs in a variety of foods, such as cheese, pears, and leafy greens. It is known to reset the circadian rhythm in humans and extend the life span in a wide variety of organisms, including yeast, worms, mice, and human cells. Some experts think it may be useful against cancer and neurodegenerative diseases.

When most people think of beneficial compounds in tomatoes, they think of **lycopene**, but the less well-known **tomatidine** may upregulate mitophagy, which is autophagy specific to the mitochondria organelles.

The native Japanese perennial **ashitaba** (*Angelica keiskei*), which belongs to the carrot family, contains a potent flavonoid called

---

132 Willcox, "Caloric Restriction, CR Mimetics, and Healthy Aging in Okinawa: Controversies and Clinical Implications," 51–58.

dimethoxychalcone, which promotes autophagy and increases longevity in lab animals and human cells in culture.[133]

One study looked at **luteolin**, a flavonoid naturally found in broccoli, celery, and parsley, and found that it activated autophagy in mice who had suffered a traumatic brain injury. The compound was neuroprotective, decreasing post-injury inflammation and swelling as well as neuron loss as a result of the injury.[134]

Two food staples of the traditional Okinawan diet are likely autophagy inducers: sea vegetables and sweet potato. Marine carotenoids, found in algae, kelp, and seaweed, contain phytochemicals that just aren't found in land plants. These include the anti-aging, anti-carcinogenic, and antioxidant **xanthophyll fucoxanthin**; the anti-carcinogenic **fucoidan**; and the anti-aging (through FOXO3 regulation) and antioxidant **astaxanthin**.[135] Sweet potato contains a protein called **sporamin**, which inhibits free radicals. It also boasts high phytonutrient content, including phenolic acids, flavonols, anthocyanins, and carotenoids.[136]

Good news for the stoner crowd: **THC**, the hallucinogenic component of marijuana, has been linked with autophagy, too. One study reported that THC killed cancer cells in both mice and—when administered intracranially (zoinks!) into two patients with recurring brain tumors—humans.[137] A recent study backs up the finding that cannabi-

133 Didac Carmona-Gutierrez et al. "The Flavonoid 4,4'-dimethoxychalcone promotes Autophagy-Dependent Longevity across Species," *Nature Communications* 10 (2019): 651. https://www.nature.com/articles/s41467-019-08555-w.

134 Jianguo Xu et al. "Posttraumatic Administration of Luteolin Protects Mice from TBI: Implication of Autophagy and Inflammation," *Brain Research* 1582 (2014): 237–46. https://doi.org/10.1016/j.brainres.2014.07.042.

135 Willcox, "Caloric Restriction, CE Mimetics, and Healthy Aging in Okinawa: Controversies and Clinical Implications," *Current Opinions in Clinical Nutrition and Metabolic Care* 17, no. 1 (2014): 51–58. https://doi.org/10.1097/MC.00000000000000019.

136 Willcox, "Caloric Restriction, CE Mimetics, and Healthy Aging in Okinawa," 51–58.

137 Maria Salazar et al. "Cannabinoid Action Induces Autophagy-Mediated Cell Death Through Stimulation of ER Stress in Human Glioma Cells," *The Journal of Clinical Investigation* 119, no. 5 (2009): 1359–72. https://doi.org/10.1172/JCI37948.

noids have an anti-tumor effect in the brain and spinal cord and calls for more research to investigate the cell mechanisms that decrease tumor growth in these cancers as well as their potential to affect other diseases of the central nervous system.[138] FYI, the 2018 study used a sativa strain.

If that's not an option, the non-hallucinogenic cannabinoid **CBD**—which is usually administered as a hemp-derived oil—has been shown to induce autophagy and disrupt inflammation in the intestines.[139]

Last but never least, at least one study has found that coffee induces autophagy in multiple tissues in mice. This effect is seen regardless of caffeine content and is likely due to its **polyphenols**.[140] Relatively high coffee consumption of 3 or 4 cups per day may also stave off cognitive decline associated with Alzheimer's disease.[141]

138   Claudia A Dumitru et al. "Cannabinoids in Glioblastoma Therapy: New Applications for Old Drugs," *Frontiers in Molecular Neuroscience* 11 (2018): 159. https://doi.org/10.3389/fnmol.2018.00159.

139   Luan C Koay et al. "Cannabinoid-Induced Autophagy Regulates Suppressor of Cytokine Signaling-3 in Intestinal Epithelium," *American Journal of Physiology* 307, no. 2 (2014): G140–48. https://doi.org/10.1152/ajpgi.00317.2013.

140   Federico Pietrocola et al. "Coffee Induces Autophagy in Vivo," *Cell Cycle* 13, no. 12 (2014): 1987–94. https://doi.org/10.4161/cc.28929.

141   Longo, *The Longevity Diet*.

CHAPTER 13

RECIPES TO BOOST AUTOPHAGY

Your options for incorporating autophagy-boosting foods into your meals are only limited by your imagination. Here are a few ideas to get you started.

BEVERAGES

TURMERIC LATTE

1 to 2 teaspoons turmeric paste*

½ cup espresso or strong coffee

½ cup milk or milk substitute

sugar or cinnamon

Melt turmeric paste into hot coffee. Froth milk and add it, along with sugar or cinnamon to taste.

*To make turmeric paste, heat ½ cup turmeric powder in 1 cup water over low heat until it thickens, about 10 minutes. Stir in ½ teaspoon black pepper and ¼ cup olive or coconut oil. Refrigerate for up to 4 weeks.

AUTOPHAGY SMOOTHIE

leafy greens, such as spinach or kale

parsley

ashitaba*

blueberries

pear chunks

frozen banana

milk or milk alternative

Combine in blender in your preferred proportions, and blend until smooth.

*Available at Asian markets/grocery stores.

SALADS

PEAR & CHEESE SALAD

leafy greens, such as spinach, kale, romaine, and arugula

pear slices

cheese slivers (such as Parmesan or aged cheddar)

olive oil

balsamic vinegar

honey

stoneground mustard

Combine the greens, pear, and cheese, and toss with olive oil and balsamic vinegar mixed with a teaspoon each of honey and stoneground mustard.

WARM BROCCOLI & TOMATO SALAD

broccoli

celery

tomatoes

pecans

parsley

olive oil

sea salt

Toss the first five ingredients in a warm pan over low heat until warmed through. Dress with olive oil and sea salt.

SEA VEGETABLE SALAD

dried seaweed or nori sheets, cut into thin strips

2 cloves garlic, minced

2 tablespoons rice vinegar

2 tablespoons soy sauce

1 tablespoon sesame oil

1 teaspoon hot chili oil (or sriracha)

carrots, shredded

cabbage, shredded

cucumber, shredded

avocado, sliced

green onions, chopped, to serve

sesame seeds, to serve

1. Rehydrate the seaweed per package directions or soak nori strips in hot water for about a minute.

2. Whisk together the garlic, vinegar, soy sauce, sesame oil, and chili oil, and toss with the seaweed, carrots, cabbage, cucumber, and avocado.

3. Top with the green onions and/or sesame seeds.

SPICY ASHITABA & SWEET POTATO SALAD

sweet potatoes, peeled, cubed, and roasted

apple chunks

celery, sliced

dried cranberries and/or blueberries

ashitaba leaves, torn

chipotles in adobo dressing*

Toss the ingredients together with desired amount of dressing.

*To make the dressing, combine 16 ounces of Greek yogurt or sour cream, 1 can of chipotles in adobo, plus a dash of salt and a dash of fresh garlic in a food processor. Process until smooth.

CHIMICHURRI-DRESSED TOMATO & PARMESAN SALAD

grape or cherry tomatoes, halved

aged Parmesan, shaved

chimichurri dressing*

Toss the tomatoes and shaved Parmesan with chimichurri dressing.

*To make the dressing, combine and blend in food processor: 1 cup of parsley leaves, 2 cloves garlic, 1 teaspoon salt, ½ teaspoon crushed red pepper, 6 tablespoons olive oil, and 1 tablespoon red wine vinegar.

ENTREES

SWEET POTATO SUSHI ROLL

sweet potato

spices

sushi rice

nori

1. Season large slivers of sweet potato as desired (maybe throw in some garlic, ginger, hot chili oil, Chinese five spice powder, or turmeric!), then bake at 350°F until cooked through (just over an hour, depending on size).

2. Roll the cooked sweet potato in sushi rice and nori, as you would an avocado roll.

TOMATO & AGED CHEESE PIE

4 large ripe tomatoes

1 teaspoon salt

piecrust (homemade or store-bought)

1½ cups aged cheese (cheddar, blue, Brie, Parmesan, Gouda, Gruyere, Swiss, or mozzarella), divided

1 teaspoon turmeric

2 cloves garlic, minced

⅓ cup fresh parsley leaves

¼ cup Greek yogurt or mayonnaise

1. Preheat the oven to 450°F.

2. Slice and salt the tomatoes and allow to drain.

3. Tuck the piecrust into a pie pan, sprinkle with ¼ cup of cheese, and bake for 10 minutes. Remove and reduce the temperature to 350°F.

4. Fill the crust with sliced tomatoes. Sprinkle with the turmeric, garlic, and parsley leaves.

5. Stir the remaining cheese into the yogurt and spread the mixture on top.

6. Bake for 30 minutes until browned.

SPICED CARROT HAND PIES

1½ pounds carrots

1 cup heavy cream

1 cup brown sugar

2 eggs

2 teaspoons ground cinnamon

½ teaspoon ground ginger

1 teaspoon vanilla extract

1 tablespoon flour

piecrust (homemade,* or store bought)

egg wash plus sugar for dusting

1. Boil the carrots until very tender, about 30 minutes.

2. Preheat the oven to 400°F.

3. Add the boiled carrots and cream to a food processor and puree. Add all the other ingredients and process.

4. Make the dough and roll it into small rounds using a biscuit cutter or mason jar lid. Scoop about a tablespoon (be careful not to overfill) of filling into rounds, fold over, and crimp edges with a fork.

5. Brush each pie with the egg wash and sprinkle with sugar.

6. Bake for about 30 minutes until golden brown.

*Piecrust from *How Sweet Eats*: In a food processor, pulse 2 cups flour, 1 tablespoon sugar, 1 teaspoon salt, and 12 tablespoons very cold butter. Add 1 egg, ½ teaspoon vinegar, and ¼ cup ice cold water and pulse until dough forms. Refrigerate 30 minutes before using.

VEGGIE NORI WRAPS WITH PEANUT SAUCE

carrots, sliced into thin, equal-sized strips

cucumber, sliced into thin, equal-sized strips

avocado, sliced into thin, equal-sized strips

bean sprouts

nori sheets

½ can full-fat coconut milk

½ cup peanut butter

3 tablespoons brown sugar

juice of ½ lime

1 tablespoon rice vinegar

3 tablespoons soy sauce

Roll the vegetables in a nori sheet, using enough vegetables to fill the wrapper. Use water to seal the edge. Whisk together all of the remaining ingredients to make a peanut dipping sauce.

SOUPS

CARROT COCONUT GINGER SOUP

1½ pounds carrots, roughly chopped

1 tablespoon olive oil, plus more to coat the carrots

1 onion, diced

3 cups water

1 can full-fat coconut milk

2 tablespoons minced fresh ginger

1 teaspoon ground cinnamon

salt and pepper, to taste

1. Preheat the oven to 450°F.

2. Coat the carrots in the olive oil and roast in the oven for about 40 minutes, turning frequently. Heat 1 tablespoon olive oil in a soup pot over medium heat. Add the onion and cook until soft.

3. Add water, carrots, coconut milk, and spices, bring to boil, then simmer for 5 minutes.

4. Puree with immersion blender or carefully puree in a traditional blender.

ROASTED PEPPER TOMATO SOUP

10 sweet mini peppers

2 pounds fresh tomatoes

2 carrots

1 onion, diced

½ cup olive oil

2 cloves garlic, minced

dash of ground cinnamon

½ cup fresh basil

1 teaspoon each salt and pepper, or to taste

6 cups water

½ cup cream (optional)

1. Preheat the oven to 400°F.

2. Add the whole peppers, tomatoes, carrots, and onion to a baking sheet. Toss with the olive oil and bake for 30 to 40 minutes, turning once, until caramelized.

3. Once they are cool enough to handle, remove the stems and seeds from the peppers and remove the skins, if preferred.

4. Add the baked veggies and all of the remaining ingredients to a soup pot and simmer for 30 minutes over medium-low heat.

5. Puree using an immersion blender (or carefully using a traditional blender). Stir in the cream, if desired.

SEAWEED MISO SOUP

4 cups water

seaweed, or 1 sheet nori

extra-firm tofu, pressed and cubed

small package mushrooms, chopped

1 teaspoon fresh garlic, or to taste

1 teaspoon fresh ginger, or to taste

¼ cup white miso

green onions, chopped

dash of chili oil (or sriracha in a pinch)

1. Add the water to a soup pot and bring to a simmer.

2. Add the seaweed (or nori in pieces), tofu, mushrooms, garlic, and ginger and cook until the mushrooms soften, about 10 minutes.

3. Whisk in the miso and cook another minute or two until just warm.

4. Top with green onions and chili oil.

DESSERTS

MINI BERRY PIES OR MINI NEXT-LEVEL (THC) BERRY PIES

6 teaspoons plain butter or chilled cannabis butter

¾ cup water

⅓ cup sugar

1 teaspoon ground cinnamon

1 tablespoon lemon juice

¼ teaspoon salt

3 tablespoons cornstarch

2½ cups blueberries, cranberries, lingonberries, or huckleberries

piecrust (homemade or store-bought)

1. Preheat the oven to 375°F.

2. Add the first seven ingredients except for 1 teaspoon of butter, to a medium saucepan and stir over medium heat.

3. Bring to a boil, then lower heat and simmer 2 to 3 minutes or until slightly thickened. Add berries and simmer another minute.

4. Prepare 12 canning jar lids with insert flipped over so that upside down lid resembles a wee pie pan. Line with piecrust.

5. Add ½ cup to ¾ cup of berry filling to each piecrust and dot with remaining teaspoon butter, broken into small bits. Enclose with more crust, venting to allow steam to escape.

6. Bake for about 15 minutes or until crust is golden brown and filling is bubbling.

EASY CANNABIS BUTTER

1¼ cups butter

½ ounce bud

4 cups water

1. Add all of the ingredients to a slow cooker and cook on low for 4 to 6 hours.

2. Strain the butter using a sieve or cheese cloth.

3. Pour boiling water over the sieved sediment, then chill the combined water and cannabis butter in the refrigerator or freezer.

4. Repeat the straining procedure so that the cannabis butter has been strained twice.

5. Scoop out the cannabis butter and rinse it under cold running water. Refrigerate for about a month or freeze for up to 6 months.

CHAPTER 14

CONCLUSION

A FINAL THOUGHT

While it is still early and new research emerges every single day in the smoking-hot field of autophagy, it is clear that this cellular process is key to enhanced life and health spans. It is also true that the research comes with big caveats that even more clinical studies are necessary, or else giddy science consumers risk oversimplifying this intensely complicated, highly regulated cell program conserved by evolution.

That said, for people reaching the age where the shiny veneer of youth is beginning to show signs of wear, or for whom family history of disease is a source of anxiety, or who already live with chronic illness, autophagy is probably the best place to look for evidence-based self-health strategies. The truth is: You are your own best advocate. All the animal studies and clinical trials in the world won't replace your personal drive to feel as good as you possibly can for as long as you possibly can. Experimenting with lifestyle changes the scientific community agrees crank up autophagy simply makes good sense.

You are probably familiar with the extremes people—maybe even your friends or family or (gulp) yourself—will go to in the pursuit of that good health. Things like cutting out entire food groups they love, building strict health regimens, or sinking massive sums of money into natural products. It's hard to scoff too hard at the weird things ancient peoples have done considering the things modern humans do for the same reason.

Renowned poet Mary Oliver once asked: "Tell me, what is it you plan to do with your one wild and precious life?" Here's hoping that chasing perfection at the expense of the good is not the message of this book. If something here resonates, give it a go; if not, please don't add that to your burden of guilt. The idea is to play around with science. Try a new food, see how fasting feels, strap on your goggles and swim more, follow some rad cell biologists on social media. And then sleep well knowing that you are indeed caring for your best, most wild and precious life.

REFERENCES

BOOKS

Hayat, M. A. "Introduction to Autophagy: Cancer, Other Pathologies, Inflammation, Immunity, Infection, and Aging." *In Autophagy*. Waltham, MA: Academic Press, 2013.

Longo, Valter. *The Longevity Diet*. New York: Avery, Penguin Group, 2018.

Whittel, Naomi. *Glow15*. Boston: Houghton Mifflin Harcourt, 2018.

Wolf, Logan. *Autophagy*. Amazon, 2018.

INTERVIEWS

Eissa (MD), N. Tony. Baylor College of Medicine, January 17, 2019.

JOURNAL ARTICLES AND WEBSITES

Alirezaei, Mehrdad et al. "Short-Term Fasting Induces Profound Neuronal Autophagy," *Autophagy* 6, no. 6 (2010): 702–710. https://doi.org/10.4161/auto.6.6.12376.

American Diabetes Association. "Statistics about Diabetes." March 22, 2018. http://www.diabetes.org/diabetes-basics/statistics/?loc=db-slabnav.

Arem, Hannah et al. "Leisure Time Physical Activity and Mortality: A Detailed Pooled Analysis of the Dose-Response Relationship." *JAMA Internal Medicine* 175, no. 6 (2015): 959–967. https://doi.org/10.1001/jamainternmed.2015.0533.

Berchem, Guy and the Laboratory of Experimental Cancer Research. Human Autophagy Database. Luxembourg Institute of Health. http://www.autophagy.lu/index.html.

Brandhorst, Sebastian et al. "A Periodic Diet That Mimics Fasting Promotes Multisystem Regeneration, Enhanced Cognitive Performance, and Health

Span." *Cell Metabolism* 22 (2015): 88–99. https://doi.org/10.1016/j.cmet .2015.05.012.

Brandt, Nina et al. "Exercise and Exercise-Training Induced Increase in Autophagy Markers in Human Skeletal Muscle." *Physiological Reports* 6, no. 7 (2018): e13651. https://doi.org/10.14814/phy2.13651.

Byun, Sanguine et al. "Therapeutic Implications of Autophagy Inducers in Immunological Disorders, Infection, and Cancer." *International Journal of Molecular Sciences* 18 (2017): 1959–1981. https://doi.org/10.3390/ ijms18091959.

Carmona-Gutierrez, Didac et al. "The Flavonoid 4,4'-Dimethoxychalcone Promotes Autophagy-Dependent Longevity Across Species." *Nature Communications* 10 (2019): 651. https://www.nature.com/articles/ s41467-019-08555-w.

Carrington, Damian. "Climate Change Could Wipe Out a Third of Parasite Species, Study Finds." *The Guardian*, September 6, 2017. https://www .theguardian.com/environment/2017/sep/06/ climate-change-could-wipe-out-a-third-of-parasite-species-study-finds.

Centers for Disease Control. "Long-Term Trends in Diabetes." April 2017. https://www.cdc.gov/diabetes/statistics/slides/long_term_trends.pdf.

Centers for Disease Control. "Parasites–Neglected Parasitic Infections." 2018 https://www.cdc.gov/parasites/npi.

Choi, In Young et al. "Nutrition and Fasting Mimicking Diets in the Prevention and Treatment of Autoimmune Diseases and Immunosenescence." *Molecular and Cellular Endocrinology* 455 (2017): 4–12. https://doi.org/10.1016/j.mce.2017.01.042.

Christian de Duve – Biographical. NobelPrize.org. Nobel Media AB 2019. Fri. 8 Mar 2019. https://www.nobelprize.org/prizes/medicine/1974/duve/ biographical.

Clarys, Peter et al. "Comparison of Nutritional Quality of the Vegan, Vegetarian, Semi-Vegetarian, Pesco-Vegetarian, and Omnivorous Diet." *Nutrients* 6, no. 3 (2014): 1318–1332. https://doi.org/10.3390/nu6031318.

Cui, Xinwen, Yiming Zhang, and Zan Wang et al. "HIIT Changes the Expression of MuRF1 and MAFBx Proteins and Proteins Involved in the mTOR

Pathway and Autophagy in Rat Skeletal Muscle." *Experimental Physiology* (2019). https://doi.org/10.1113/EP087601.

Dlugonska, Henryka. "Autophagy as a Universal Intracellular Process. A Comment on the 2016 Nobel Prize in Physiology or Medicine." *Annals of Parasitology* 63, no. 3 (2017): 153–157. https://doi.org/10.17420/ap6303 .100.

Drye, Willie. "Fountain of Youth." *National Geographic*. Accessed January 16, 2019. https://www.nationalgeographic.com/archaeology-and-history/ archaeology/fountain-of-youth.

Dumitru, Claudia A. et al. "Cannabinoids in Glioblastoma Therapy: New Applications for Old Drugs." *Frontiers in Molecular Neuroscience* 11 (2018): 159. https://doi.org/10.3389/fnmol.2018.00159.

Fan, Jingjing et al. "Spermidine Coupled with Exercise Rescues Skeletal Muscle Atrophy." *Oncotarget* 8, no. 11 (2017): 17475–17490. https://doi .org/10.18632/oncotarget.15728.

Finkbeiner, Steven. "The Autophagy Lysosomal Pathway and Neuro-degeneration." *Cold Spring Harbor Perspectives in Biology*. https://doi.org/ 10.1101/cshperspect.a033993.

Frake, Rebecca A. et al. "Autophagy and Neurodegeneration." *Journal of Clinical Investigation* 125, no. 1 (2015): 65–74. https://doi.org/10.1172/ JCI73944.

Garatachea, Nuria et al. "Exercise Attentuates the Major Hallmarks of Aging." *Rejuvenation Research* 18, no. 1 (2015): 57–89. https://doi.org/ 10.1089/rej.2014.1623.

Gelino, Sara et al. "Intestinal Autophagy Improves Healthspan and Longevity in C. Elegans during Dietary Restriction." *PLOS Genetics* 12, no. 7 (2017): e1006135. https://doi.org/10.1371/journal.pgen.1006135.

Guo, Y., X. Zhang, and T. Wu et al. "Autophagy in Skin Diseases." *Dermatology* 235, no. 5 (2019): 380–89. https://doi.org/10.1159/000500470.

Harnett, Margaret M. et al. "From Christian de Duve to Yoshinori Ohsumi: More to Autophagy than Just Dining at Home." *Biomedical Journal* 40 (2017): 9–22. https://doi.org/ 10.1016/j.bj.2016.12.004.

Hartman, Adam L. and Eileen P. G. Vining. "Clinical Aspects of the Ketogenic Diet." *Epilepsia* 48, no. 1 (2007): 31–42. https://doi.org/10.1111/j.1528-1167 .2007.00914.x.

Harvard School of Public Health. "The Nutrition Source: Protein." https:// www.hsph.harvard.edu/nutritionsource/what-should-you-eat/protein.

Harvie, Michell N. and Tony Howell. "Could Intermittent Energy Restriction and Intermittent Fasting Reduce Rates of Cancer in Obese, Overweight, and Normal-Weight Subjects? A Summary of Evidence." *Advances in Nutrition* 7 (2016): 690–705. https://doi.org/10.3945/an.115.011767.

He C. et al. *Nature* 481, no. 7382 (2012): 1476–4687. https://doi.org/ 10.1038/nature10758.

Hornyak, Tim. "The Rise and Rise of a Biology Superstar." *Nature Index* (2017): S19.

HUGO Gene Nomenclature Committee. Autophagy-related gene group. https://www.genenames.org/data/genegroup/#!/group/1022.

Huseby, Carol J. et al. "The Role of Annealing and Fragmentation in Human Tau Aggregation Dynamics." *Journal of Biological Chemistry* 294, no. 13 (2019): 4728–4737. https://doi.org/10.1074/jbc.RA118.006943.

Ke, Po-Yuan. "Horning Cell Self-Digestion: Autophagy Wins the 2016 Nobel Prize in Physiology or Medicine." *Biomedical Journal* 40, no. 1 (2017): 5–8. https://doi.org/ 10.1016/j.bj.2017.03.003.

Kim, Hei Sung, Seo-Yeon Park, Seok Hoon Moon et al. "Autophagy in Human Skin Fibroblasts: Impact of Age." *International Journal of Molecular Sciences* 19, no. 8 (2018): 2254. https://doi.org/10.3390/ijms19082254.

Kim, J. et al. "The Role of Autophagy in Systemic Metabolism and Human-Type Diabetes." *Molecules and Cells* 41, no. 1 (2018): 11–17. https://doi. org/10.14348/molcells.2018.2228.

Koay, Luan C. et al. "Cannabinoid-Induced Autophagy Regulates Suppressor of Cytokine Signaling-3 in Intestinal Epithelium." *American Journal of Physiology* 307, no. 2 (2014): G140–G148. https://doi.org/10.1152/ ajpgi.00317.2013.

Kroemer, Guido. "Autophagy: A Druggable Process That Is Deregulated in Aging and Human Disease." *Journal of Clinical Investigation* 125, no. 1 (2015): 1–4. https://doi.org/10.1172/JCI78652.

Levine, Morgan E. et al. "Low Protein Intake Is Associated with a Major Reduction in Igf-1, Cancer, and Overall Mortality in the 65 and Younger But Not Older Population." *Cell Metabolism* 19, no. 3 (2014) : 407–417. https://doi.org/10.1016/j.cmet.2014.02.006.

Li, Fang-Hui, Lei Sun, and Da-Shuai Wu et al. "Proteomics-Based Identification of Different Training Adaptations of Aged Skeletal Muscle Following Long-Term High-Intensity Interval and Moderate-Intensity Continuous Training in Aged Rats." *Aging* 11, no. 12 (2019): 4159–4182. https://doi.org/10.18632/aging.102044

Li, Fang-Hui, Tao Li, and Jing-Yi Ai et al. "Beneficial Autophagic Activities, Mitochondrial Function, and Metabolic Phenotype Adaptations Promoted by High-Intensity Interval Training in a Rat Model." *Frontiers in Physiology* 9 (2018): 571. https://doi.org/10.3389/fphys.2018.00571.

Live Science. "Germs Really Are Everywhere [infographic]." Live Science website. October 31, 2011. https://www.livescience.com/16787-germs-everyday-surfaces-infographic.html.

Longo, Valter D. and Satchidananda Panda. "Fasting, Circadian Rhythms, and Time Restricted Feeding in Healthy Life Span." *Cell Metabolism* 23, no. 6 (2016): 1048–59. https://doi.org/10.1016/j.cmet.2016.06.001.

Lopez-Otin, Carlos et al. "The Hallmarks of Aging." *Cell* 153 (2013): 1194–17. https://doi.org/10.1016/j.cell.2013.05.039.

Madeo, Frank et al. "Essential Role for Autophagy in Life Span Extension." *Journal of Clinical Investigation* 125, no. 1 (2015): 85–93. https://doi.org/10.1172/JCI73946.

Maiuri, Maria Chiara and Guido Kroemer. "Therapeutic Modulation of Autophagy: Which Disease Comes First?" *Cell Death and Differentiation* 26 (2019): 680–89. https://doi.org/10.1038/s41418-019-0290-0.

Matthews, Susan E. "Why Your Cell Phone Has More Bacteria Than a Toilet Seat." *Live Science*. August 30, 2012. https://www.livescience.com/22822-cell-phones-germs.html.

Mattison, Julie A. et al. "Caloric Restriction Improves Health and Survival of Rhesus Monkeys." *Nature Communications* 8, no 14063 (2016). https://doi.org/10.1038/ncomms14063.

Mattson, Mark P. et al. "Impact of Intermittent Fasting on Health and Disease Processes." *Ageing Research Review* 39 (2017): 46–58. https://doi.org/10.1016/j.arr.2016.10.005.

Mayo Clinic. "Diabetes and Alzheimer's Linked." April 19, 2019. https://www.mayoclinic.org/diseases-conditions/alzheimers-disease/in-depth/diabetes-and-alzheimers/ART-20046987.

Mizushima, Noboru and Masaaki Komatsu. "Autophagy: Renovation of Cells and Tissues." *Cell* 147 (2011): 728–41. https://doi.org/10.1016/j.cell.2011.10.026.

Nakamura, Shuhei and Tamotsu Yoshimori. "Autophagy and Longevity." *Molecules and Cells* 41, no. 1 (2018): 65–72. https://doi.org/10.14348/molcells.2018.2333.

National Institute on Aging. "Calorie Restriction and Fasting Diets: What Do We Know?" National Institutes of Health. (2018) www.nia.nih.gov/health/calorie-restriction-and-fasting-diets-what-do-we-know.

National Institutes of Health. "Estimates of Funding for Various Research, Condition, and Disease Categories." US Department of Health and Human Services, April 19, 2019. https://report.nih.gov/categorical_spending.aspx.

National Institutes of Health, Genetics Home Reference. "What Is a gene?" US Department of Health and Human Services, May 14, 2019. https://ghr.nlm.nih.gov/primer/basics/gene.

Ohsumi, Yoshinori. "Historical Landmarks of Autophagy Research." *Cell Research* 24 (2014): 9–23. https://doi.org/10.1038/cr.2013.169.

Oczypok, Elizabeth A. et al. "It's a Cell-Eat-Cell World: Autophagy and Phagocytosis." *The American Journal of Pathology* 182, no. 3 (2013): 612–22. https://doi.org/10.1016/j.ajpath.2012.12.017.

Park, Seo-Yeon, Eun Byun, and Jeong Lee et al. "Air Pollution, Autophagy, and Skin Aging: Impact of Particulate Matter (PM_{10}) on Human Dermal Fibroblasts." *International Journal of Molecular Sciences* 19, no. 9 (2018): 2727. https://doi.org/10.3390/ijms19092727.

Pietrocola, Federico et al. "Coffee Induces Autophagy in Vivo." *Cell Cycle* 13, no. 12 (2014): 1987–94. https://doi.org/10.4161/cc.28929.

Puleston, Daniel and Anna Katharina Simon. "Autophagy in the Immune System." *Immunology* 141, no. 1 (2014): 1–8. https://doi.org/10.1111/imm.12165.

Rangan, P. et al. "Fasting-Mimicking Diet Modulates Microbiota and Promotes Intestinal Regeneration to Reduce Inflammatory Bowel Disease Pathology." *Cell Reports* 26, no. 10 (2019): 2704–2719. https://doi.org/10.1016/j.celrep.2019.02.019.

Rocchi, Altea and Congcong He. "Activating Autophagy by Aerobic Exercise in Mice." *Journal of Visualized Experiments* 120 (2017): e55099. https://doi.org/10.3791/55099.

Rubinsztein, David C. et al. "Autophagy and Aging." *Cell* 146 (2011): 682–95. https://doi.org/10.1016/j.cell.2011.07.030.

Salazar, Maria et al. "Cannabinoid Action Induces Autophagy-Mediated Cell Death Through Stimulation of ER Stress in Human Glioma Cells." *The Journal of Clinical Investigation* 119, no. 5 (2009): 1359–72. https://doi.org/10.1172/JCI37948.

Shetty, Ashok K. et al. "Emerging Anti-aging Strategies—Scientific Basis and Efficacy." *Aging and Disease* 9, no. 6 (2018): 1165–84. https://doi.org/10.14336/AD.2018.1026.

Tooze, Sharon A. and Ivan Dikic. "Autophagy Captures the Nobel Prize." *Cell* 167 (2016): 1433–35. https://doi.org/10.1016/j.cell.2016.11.023.

Udristioiu, Aurelian and Delia Nica-Badea. "Autophagy Dysfunctions Associated with Cancer Cells and Their Therapeutic Implications." *Biomedicine & Pharmacotherapy* 115 (2019): 108892. https://doi.org/10.1016/j.biopha.2019.108892.

Vainshtein, Anna and David A. Hood. "The Regulation of Autophagy During Exercise in Skeletal Muscle." *Journal of Applied Physiology* 120, no. 6 (2016): 664–73. https://doi.org/10.1152/japplphysiol.00550.2015.

Wang, Y., Xiang Wen, and Dan Hao et al. "Insights into Autophagy Machinery in Cells Related to Skin Diseases and Strategies for Therapeutic Modulation." *Biomedicine & Pharmacotherapy* 113 (2019): 108775. https://doi.org/10.1016/j.biopha.2019.108775

Whitcomb, David C. "What Is Personalized Medicine and What Should It Replace?" *National Reviews in Gastroenterology and Hepatology* 9, no. 7 (2012): 418–24. https://doi.org/10.1038/nrgastro.2012.100.

Willcox, Bradley J. and Donald Craig Willcox. "Caloric Restriction, CR Mimetics, and Healthy Aging in Okinawa: Controversies and Clinical Implications." *Current Opinions in Clinical Nutrition and Metabolic Care* 17, no. 1 (2014): 51–8. https://doi.org/10.1097/MC.00000000000000019.

Xu, Jianguo et al. "Posttraumatic Administration of Luteolin Protects Mice From TBI: Implication of Autophagy and Inflammation." *Brain Research* 1582 (2014): 237–46. https://doi.org/10.1016/j.brainres.2014.07.042.

Yang, Zhen et al. "Autophagy in Autoimmune Disease." *Journal of Molecular Medicine (Berlin, Germany)* 93, no. 7 (2015): 707–17. https://doi.org/10.1007/s00109-015-1297-8.

"Yoshinori Ohsumi Biographical." *The Nobel Prizes 2016*. Sagamore Beach: Science History Publications, a division of Watson Publishing International LLC, 2017.

"Yoshinori Ohsumi Banquet Speech." *The Nobel Prizes 2016*. https://www.nobelprize.org/prizes/medicine/2016/ohsumi/25025-yoshinori-ohsumi-banquet-speech-2016.

Yutin, Natalya et al. "The Origins of Phagocytosis and Eukaryogenesis." *Biology Direct* 4, no. 9 (2009). https://doi.org/10.1186/1745-6150-4-9.

CONVERSIONS

COMMON CONVERSIONS

1 gallon = 4 quarts = 8 pints = 16 cups = 128 fluid ounces = 3.8 liters
1 quart = 2 pints = 4 cups = 32 ounces = .95 liter
1 pint = 2 cups = 16 ounces = 480 ml
1 cup = 8 ounces = 240 ml
¼ cup = 4 tablespoons = 12 teaspoons = 2 ounces = 60 ml

TEMPERATURE CONVERSIONS

FAHRENHEIT (°F)	CELSIUS (°C)
200°F	95°C
225°F	110°C
250°F	120°C
275°F	135°C
300°F	150°C
325°F	165°C
350°F	175°C
375°F	190°C
400°F	200°C
425°F	220°C
450°F	230°C
475°F	245°C

VOLUME CONVERSIONS

US	U.S. EQUIVALENT	METRIC
1 tablespoon (3 teaspoons)	½ fluid ounce	15 milliliters
¼ cup	2 fluid ounces	60 milliliters
⅓ cup	3 fluid ounces	80 milliliters
½ cup	4 fluid ounces	120 milliliters
⅔ cup	5 fluid ounces	160 milliliters
¾ cup	6 fluid ounces	180 milliliters
1 cup	8 fluid ounces	240 milliliters
2 cups	16 fluid ounces	480 milliliters

WEIGHT CONVERSIONS

US	METRIC
½ ounce	15 grams
1 ounce	30 grams
2 ounces	60 grams
¼ pound	115 grams
⅓ pound	150 grams
½ pound	225 grams
¾ pound	340 grams
1 pound	450 grams

INDEX

ACKNOWLEDGMENTS

This book could not have happened without the tireless work of my wife, Bobbi Mayer, who wrangled our small children on nights and weekends, made beautiful food and endless cups of coffee appear on my desk, and who makes me believe I can do things. Thank you for boldly reaching over my shoulder and hitting "send" on that first piece of science writing that I was too scared to submit a decade ago. I'm so glad you moved in next door and swept me off my feet.

Thank you to Addison, who clocked a million hours babysitting his sisters while I read and interviewed and typed words. Being your parent and friend is a delight. And, of course, thank you to Sonora and Xochitl, who gave me time to work and reminded me that writing can't be that serious since Peppa's Mummy does it just fine—and she's a pig.

I'm grateful to the team at Ulysses—particularly Bridget Thoreson and Renee Rutledge—for conceiving the idea for this book, selecting me to write it, and editing it. And I'm indebted to the network of women and genderqueer writers and editors who have been a reservoir of collective wisdom and community.

I feel so lucky to have the fun job of rolling around in PubMed, hunting and reading and piecing together the ideas represented by the vast catalog of research out there. Hopefully it's obvious that I think the researchers devoting their careers to unraveling the science—and who take the time to talk with science writers like me and send us their work and their connections—are the heroes of this story.

ABOUT THE AUTHOR

Melissa Mayer is a science writer who regularly covers cell biology and neuroscience. She earned a degree from Trinity University and biology teaching credentials from the University of Texas at San Antonio. She spent 10 years as a classroom teacher and 5 years as a science blogger reporting proteomics and genomics in the biotech space before expanding to cover science more broadly. Her work has appeared in *Mental Floss*, the Society for Neuroscience, the Entomological Society of America, and *Bitch* media, among others. She also wrote *Coping with Date Rape and Acquaintance Rape*, *Why We Rage: The Science of Anger*, and *Why We Worry: The Science of Anxiety* (Decoding the Mind series).